This book is dedicated to
Wendy
Jim and Maeve
Sally, Garrie, Samuel and Gregory
Robert and Tracey

Acquisitions editor: Heidi Allen
Development editor: Robert Edwards
Desk editor: Jane Campbell
Production Controller: Chris Jarvis
Cover designer: Greg Harris

Gait Analysis: an introduction

Third Edition

Michael W. Whittle

Walter M. Cline Chair of Excellence in Rehabilitation Technology
The University of Tennessee at Chattanooga
Chattanooga, Tennessee, USA

and

Director
H. Carey Hanlin Motion Analysis Laboratory
The University of Tennessee at Chattanooga
Chattanooga, Tennessee, USA

formerly

Acting Director
Oxford Orthopaedic Engineering Centre
University of Oxford
Oxford, UK

EDINBURGH LONDON NEW YORK OXFORD
PHILADELPHIA ST LOUIS SYDNEY TORONTO 1996

Butterworth-Heinemann
An imprint of Elsevier Science Limited
Robert Stevenson House,
1-3 Baxter's Place,
Leith Walk,
Edinburgh
EH1 3AF

First published in Great Britain 1990
First edition 1990
Second edition 1996
Reprinted 1997
Third edition 2002
Reprinted 2003 (twice)

British Library Cataloguing in Publication Data
Whittle, Michael
  Gait analysis: an introduction. - 3rd ed.
  1. Gait in humans   2. Gait disorders
  I. Title
  612.7'6

Library of Congress Cataloging in Publication Data
[copy to come]

ISBN 0 7506 5262 4

Typeset by David Gregson Associates, Beccles, Suffolk
Printed and bound in Great Britain by Martins the Printers, Berwick upon Tweed

ELSEVIER
SCIENCE

your source for books,
journals and multimedia
in the health sciences
www.elsevierhealth.com

Contents

Preface to third edition

Gait analysis is the systematic study of human walking, using the eye and brain of experienced observers, augmented by instrumentation for measuring body movements and body mechanics and the activity of the muscles. In individuals with conditions affecting their ability to walk, gait analysis may be used to make detailed diagnoses and to plan optimal treatment.

Over the past few years gait analysis has 'come of age', and in a number of centers it is now used routinely to provide the best possible care for certain groups of patients – most notably those with cerebral palsy. Since the benefits of this approach have been well established, it is to be hoped that its usage will continue to spread, so that many more will benefit from the better treatment decisions that can be made when gait analysis is used.

I am happy to believe that the first two editions of this book have contributed to this process by providing a text that does not require a high level of academic learning to be understood. I have heard from people all over the world that they have found the book useful, and this I find very gratifying.

The next stage in the evolution of gait analysis will hopefully involve improvements in the ease and speed with which gait data can be collected and interpreted, and decreases in the cost of the equipment and the skill level needed to use it. Significant strides have been made in all of these aspects since the second edition of the book was published in 1996, but there is clearly still room for improvement.

The inclusion of a CD-ROM with 'real' gait data with this book will, it is hoped, provide the reader with a better opportunity to get a feel for this fascinating subject.

Michael W. Whittle
Chattanooga, Tennessee
May 2001

Preface to first edition

Gait analysis is the systematic study of human walking. It is often helpful in the medical management of those diseases which affect the locomotor system. Over the past few years, there has been an increasing interest in the subject, particularly among practitioners and students of physical therapy, bio-engineering, and several branches of medicine, including orthopedics, rheumatology, neurology and rehabilitation. Most previous books on the subject have been written for specialists, and are thus unsuitable for the student or general reader, since they assumed a certain amount of previous knowledge of the subject. I have attempted to write an introductory textbook, with the aim of providing the reader with a solid grounding in the subject, but without assuming a particular background or level of prior knowledge.

Chapter 1 is devoted to the basic sciences underlying gait analysis – anatomy, physiology, and biomechanics. It is intended to give the reader who is new to these subjects the minimum required to make sense of gait analysis. It should also provide a refresher course for those who have once had such knowledge but forgotten it, as well as being a convenient source of reference material. Chapters 2 and 3 deal with normal gait and pathological gait respectively, showing the remarkable efficiency of the normal walking process, and the various ways in which it may be affected by disease. Chapter 4 is devoted to methods of measurement, pointing out that gait analysis does not have to be difficult or expensive, but that the more complicated systems provide detailed information which cannot be obtained in any other way. The final chapter, Chapter 5, deals with the applications of gait analysis. This is the area in which the most progress has been made in the past few years, and in which the most progress is to be anticipated in the future. The literature of the field is heavily biased towards research rather than clinical application, but the value of the methodology is gradually coming to be realized in a number of clinical conditions.

I have deliberately avoided giving references to theses and conference proceedings, since these may be difficult to find. Chapter 1 contains no references at all, as everything in it should be easy to find in standard textbooks. I have restricted the number of references quoted in the remainder of the book, not through ignorance of laziness, but rather in an attempt to identify only the most important references on particular topics. These will in turn lead on to other references, should the reader wish to study that topic in greater depth. Those not familiar with it should ask their librarian about the Science Citation Index, which uses key references from the past to identify more recent publications in the same field.

I have use Système International (SI) units throughout this book. I make no apology for this – everyone working in this field should be using the measurement units of science, rather than those of the grocery store! However, conversions are given in Appendix 2.

Since the origins of this book are international, it is hoped that it will appeal to an international readership. It was written during my last few months at the University of Oxford, England, and my first few months at the University of Tennessee at Chattanooga, in the USA. It draws on reference material from both sides of the Atlantic, and parts of it were written on journeys across that ocean!

Michael W. Whittle
Chattanooga, Tennessee
May 1990

Acknowledgements

I would particularly like to thank my wife Wendy for her encouragement, support and tolerance while I have been preparing this book. Particular thanks are also due to Karen Hood, Jeannette Beach and Locke Davis, who work with me in the gait laboratory and have taught me so much about clinical gait analysis. The CD-ROM that accompanies this book contains data generously supplied by James Carollo and Nancy Denniston, from The Children's Hospital, Denver and some text written by Chris Kirtley. The Polygon computer program used to prepare the interactive multimedia presentation of gait was provided through the generosity of Vicon Motion Systems Ltd. Three other groups have also contributed in different ways to this book – my faculty colleagues, the students I teach, and the patients we have seen in the laboratory. I would finally like to thank the administrators of The University of Tennessee at Chattanooga and of the Siskin Hospital for Physical Rehabilitation, Chattanooga, for their support.

Basic sciences

All voluntary movement, including walking, results from a complicated process involving the brain, spinal cord, peripheral nerves, muscles, bones and joints. Before considering in detail the process of walking, what can go wrong with it, and how it can be studied, it is necessary to have a basic understanding of three scientific disciplines – anatomy, physiology and biomechanics. It is hoped that this chapter will provide the rudiments of these subjects for those not already familiar with them, will review the topic for those who are, and will also provide a convenient source of reference material.

Anatomy

It is not the intention of this book to attempt to teach in detail the anatomy of the locomotor system, which is well covered in several other books (e.g. Palastanga *et al.*, 1989). The notes that follow give only an outline of the subject, but one that should be sufficient for an understanding of gait analysis. The anatomical names for the different parts of the body vary somewhat from one textbook to another; as far as possible the most common name has been used. The section starts by describing some basic anatomical terms, and then goes on to describe the bones, joints, muscles and nervous system. Although the arteries and veins are essential to the functioning of the locomotor system they will not be described here, since they generally affect gait only indirectly, through their role in providing oxygen and nutrients for the nerves and muscles, and removing waste products.

Basic anatomical terms

The anatomical terms describing the relationships between different parts of the body are based on the *anatomical position*, in which a person is standing upright with the feet together and the arms by the sides of the body, with the palms forward. This position, together with the reference

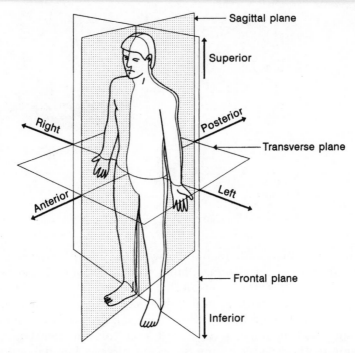

Figure 1.1 The anatomical position, with three reference planes and six fundamental directions.

planes and the terms describing relationships between different parts of the body, is illustrated in Fig. 1.1.

Six terms are used to describe directions, with relation to the center of the body. These are best defined by example:

1. The umbilicus is *anterior*
2. The buttocks are *posterior*
3. The head is *superior*
4. The feet are *inferior*
5. *Left* is self-evident
6. So is *right*.

The anterior surface of the body is *ventral* and the posterior surface is *dorsal*. The word *dorsum* is used for both the back of the hand and the upper surface of the foot. The terms *cephalad* (towards the head) and *caudad* (towards the 'tail') are sometimes used in place of superior and inferior.

Within a single part of the body, six additional terms are used to describe relationships:

1. *Medial* means towards the midline of the body: the big toe is on the medial side of the foot
2. *Lateral* means away from the midline of the body: the little toe is on the lateral side of the foot
3. *Proximal* means towards the rest of the body: the shoulder is the proximal part of the arm

Figure 1.2 Movements about the hip joint (above) and knee joint (below).

4. *Distal* means away from the rest of the body: the fingers are the distal part of the hand
5. *Superficial* structures are close to the surface
6. *Deep* structures are far from the surface.

The motion of the limbs is described using reference planes:

1. A *sagittal* plane is any plane that divides part of the body into right and left portions; the *median* plane is the midline sagittal plane, which divides the whole body into right and left halves
2. A *frontal* plane divides a body part into front and back portions
3. A *transverse* plane divides a body part into upper and lower portions.

The term *coronal plane* is equivalent to frontal plane, and the transverse plane may also be called the *horizontal plane*, although it is only horizontal when in the standing position.

Most joints can only move in one or two of these three planes. The directions of these motions for the hip and knee are shown in Fig. 1.2, and for the ankle and foot in Fig. 1.3. The possible movements are:

1. *Flexion* and *extension*, which take place in the sagittal plane; in the ankle these movements are called *dorsiflexion* and *plantarflexion*, respectively
2. *Abduction* and *adduction*, which take place in the frontal plane
3. *Internal* and *external rotation*, which take place in the transverse plane; they are also called *medial* and *lateral* rotation, respectively, the term referring to the motion of the anterior surface.

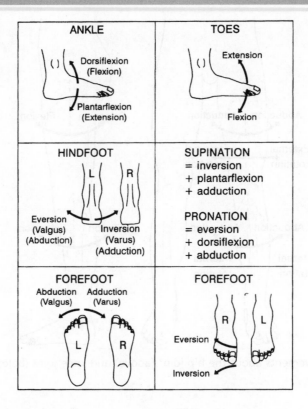

Figure 1.3 Movements of the ankle, toes, hindfoot and forefoot.

Other terms that are used to describe the motions of the joints or body segments are:

1. *Varus* and *valgus*, which describe an angulation of a joint towards or away from the midline, respectively; knock knees are in valgus, bow legs are in varus
2. *Pronation* and *supination*, which are rotations about the long axis of the forearm or foot; pronation of both hands brings the thumbs together, supination brings the little fingers together (*aide memoire*: you can hold *soup* in your hands if the palms are upwards)
3. *Inversion* of the feet brings the soles together; *eversion* causes the soles to point away from the midline.

Terminology in the foot is often confusing and lacking in standardization. This book has adopted what is probably the commonest convention (Fig. 1.3), in which the term pronation is used for a combined movement that consists primarily of eversion but also includes some dorsiflexion and forefoot abduction. Similarly, supination is primarily inversion but also includes some plantarflexion and forefoot adduction. These movements represent a 'twisting' of the forefoot relative to the hindfoot. However, some authorities regard pronation and supination as the basic movements, and eversion and inversion as the combined movements.

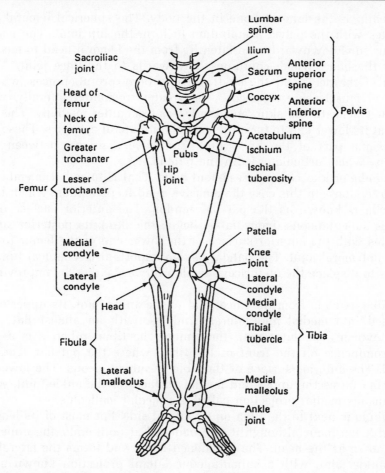

Figure 1.4 Bones and joints of the lower limbs.

Bones

It could be argued that almost every bone in the body takes part in walking. However, from a practical point of view it is generally only necessary to consider the bones of the pelvis and legs. These are shown in Fig. 1.4.

The *pelvis* is formed from the sacrum, the coccyx and the two innominate bones. The *sacrum* consists of the five sacral vertebrae, fused together. The *coccyx* is the vestigial 'tail', made of three to five rudimentary vertebrae. The *innominate bone* on each side is formed by the fusion of three bones – the *ilium*, *ischium* and *pubis*. The only real movement between the bones of the pelvis occurs at the sacroiliac joint, and this movement is generally very small in adults. It is thus reasonable, for the purposes of gait analysis, to regard the pelvis as being a single rigid structure. The superior surface of the sacrum articulates with the fifth lumbar vertebra of the spine. On each side of the lower part of the pelvis is the acetabulum, which is the proximal part of the hip joint, being the socket into which the head of the femur fits.

The *femur* is the longest bone in the body. The spherical femoral head articulates with the pelvic acetabulum to form the hip joint. The neck of the femur runs downwards and laterally from the femoral head to meet the shaft of the bone, which continues downwards to the knee joint. At the junction of the neck and the shaft are two bony protuberances, where a number of muscles are inserted – the greater trochanter laterally, which can be felt beneath the skin, and the lesser trochanter medially. The bone widens at its lower end to form the medial and lateral condyles. These form the proximal part of the knee joint, and have a groove between them anteriorly, which articulates with the patella.

The *patella* or kneecap is a sesamoid bone. That is to say, it is embedded within a tendon – in this case the massive quadriceps tendon, which below the patella is known as the patellar tendon. The anterior surface of the patella is subcutaneous (immediately below the skin); its posterior surface articulates with the anterior surface of the lower end of the femur to form the patellofemoral joint. The patella has an important mechanical function, which is to displace the quadriceps tendon forwards, thereby improving its leverage.

The *tibia* extends from the knee joint to the ankle joint. Its upper end is broadened into medial and lateral condyles, with an almost flat upper surface, which articulates with the femur. The tibial tubercle is a small bony prominence on the front of the tibia, where the patellar tendon is inserted. The anterior surface of the tibia is subcutaneous. The lower end of the tibia forms the upper and medial surfaces of the ankle joint, with a subcutaneous medial projection called the medial malleolus.

The *fibula* is next to the tibia on its lateral side. For most of its length it is a fairly slim bone, although it is broadened at both ends, the upper end being known as the head. The broadened lower end forms the lateral part of the ankle joint, with a subcutaneous lateral projection known as the lateral malleolus. The tibia and fibula are in contact with each other at their upper and lower ends, as the tibiofibular joints. Movements at these joints are very small, and will not be considered further. A layer of fibrous tissue known as the interosseous membrane lies between the bones.

The foot is a very complicated structure (Fig. 1.5) which is best thought of as being in three parts:

1. The *hindfoot*, which consists of two bones, one on top of the other
2. The *midfoot*, which consists of five bones packed closely together
3. The *forefoot*, which consists of the five metatarsals and the toes.

The *talus* or astragalus is the upper of the two bones in the hindfoot. Its superior surface forms the ankle joint, articulating above and medially with the tibia, and laterally with the fibula. Below, the talus articulates with the calcaneus through the subtalar joint. It articulates anteriorly with the most medial and superior of the midfoot bones – the navicular.

The *calcaneus* or os calcis lies below the talus, and articulates with it through the subtalar joint. Its lower surface transmits the body weight to the ground through a thick layer of fat, fibrous tissue and skin – the heelpad. The anterior surface articulates with the most lateral and inferior of the midfoot bones – the cuboid.

Figure 1.5 Bones of the right foot, seen from above.

The midfoot consists of five bones:

1. The *navicular*, which is medial and superior
2. The *cuboid*, which is lateral and inferior
3. Three *cuneiform* bones (medial, intermediate and lateral), which lie in a row, distal to the navicular.

The five *metatarsals* lie roughly parallel to each other, the lateral two articulating with the cuboid and the medial three with the three cuneiform bones.

The *phalanges* are the bones of the toes; there are two in the big toe and three in each of the other toes. The big toe is also called the great toe or *hallux*.

Joints and ligaments

A joint occurs where one bone is in contact with another. From a practical point of view, they can be divided into synovial joints, in which significant movement can take place, and the various other types of joint, in which only small movements can occur. Since gait analysis is normally only concerned with fairly large movements, the description that follows deals only with *synovial joints*. In a *synovial joint* the bone ends are covered in *cartilage* and the joint is surrounded by a *synovial capsule*, which secretes the lubricant *synovial fluid*. Most joints are stabilized by *ligaments*, which are bands of relatively inelastic fibrous tissue connecting one bone to another. *Fascia* is a special type of ligament, being a continuous sheet of fibrous tissue.

The *hip* joint is the only true ball-and-socket joint in the body, the ball being the head of the femur and the socket the acetabulum of the pelvis. Extremes of movement are prevented by a number of ligaments running between the pelvis and the femur, by a capsule surrounding the joint, and by a small ligament – the ligamentum teres – which joins the center of the head of the femur to the center of the acetabulum. The joint is capable of flexion, extension, abduction, adduction, internal and external rotation (Fig. 1.2).

The *knee* joint consists of the medial and lateral condyles of the femur, above, and the corresponding condyles of the tibia, below. The articular surfaces on the medial and lateral sides are separate, making the knee joint, in effect, two joints, side by side. The femoral condyles are curved both from front to back and from side to side, whereas the tibial condyles are almost flat. The gap this would leave around the point of contact is filled, on each side, by a meniscus, commonly called a cartilage, which acts to spread the load and reduce the pressure at the point of contact.

The motion of the joint is controlled by five ligaments that between them exert very close control over the movements of the knee:

1. The medial collateral ligament (MCL), which prevents the medial side of the joint from opening up (i.e. it opposes abduction or valgus)
2. The lateral collateral ligament (LCL), which similarly opposes adduction or varus
3. The posterior joint capsule, which prevents hyperextension (excessive extension) of the joint
4. The anterior cruciate ligament (ACL), found in the center of the joint, between the condyles; this is attached to the tibia anteriorly and the femur posteriorly, prevents the tibia from moving forwards relative to the femur, and also helps to prevent excessive rotation
5. The posterior cruciate ligament (PCL), also in the center of the joint; this is attached to the tibia posteriorly and the femur anteriorly, prevents the tibia from moving backwards relative to the femur, and also helps to limit rotation.

The anterior and posterior cruciate ligaments are named for the positions in which they are attached to the tibia. They appear to act together as what engineers call a four-bar-linkage, which imposes a combination of sliding and rolling on the joint, and moves the contact point forwards as the joint extends and backwards as it flexes. This means that the axis about which the joint flexes and extends is not fixed, but changes with the angle of flexion or extension.

In the normal individual the motions of the knee are flexion and extension, with a small amount of internal and external rotation. Significant amounts of abduction and adduction are only seen in damaged knees. As the knee comes to full extension, there is an external rotation of a few degrees – the so-called automatic rotation or 'screw-home' mechanism.

The *patellofemoral* joint lies between the posterior surface of the patella and the anterior surface of the femur. The articular surface consists of a shallow V-shaped ridge on the patella, which fits into a shallow groove between the medial and lateral condyles. The principal movement is the patella gliding up and down in this groove during extension and flexion of the knee respectively. This causes different areas of the patella to come into contact with different parts of the joint surfaces of the femur. There is also some medial–lateral movement of the patella.

The *ankle* or talocrural joint has three surfaces – upper, medial and lateral. The upper surface is the main articulation of the joint; it is cylindrical, and formed by the tibia above and the talus below. The medial joint surface is between the talus and the inner aspect of the medial malleolus of the tibia. Correspondingly, the lateral joint surface is between the talus and the inner surface of the lateral malleolus of the fibula.

The major ligaments of the ankle joint are those between the tibia and the fibula, which prevent these two bones from moving apart, and the collateral ligaments on both sides between the two malleoli and both the talus and calcaneus, which keep the joint surfaces in contact. The ankle joint, being cylindrical, has only one significant type of motion – dorsiflexion and plantarflexion, corresponding to flexion and extension in other joints.

The *subtalar* or talocalcaneal joint lies between the talus above and the calcaneus below. It has three articular surfaces; two anterior and medial, and one posterior and lateral. Large numbers of ligaments join the two bones to each other and to all the adjacent bones. The axis of the joint is oblique, running primarily forwards, but also upwards and medially. From a functional point of view the importance of the subtalar joint is that it permits abduction and adduction (valgus/varus motion) of the hindfoot. When performing gait analysis it is usually impossible to distinguish between movement at the ankle joint and that taking place at the subtalar joint, and it is reasonable to refer to motion taking place at the 'ankle/subtalar complex'. This motion in normal individuals includes dorsiflexion, plantarflexion, hindfoot abduction and hindfoot adduction, plus a small amount of rotation about the long axis of the leg.

The *midtarsal* joints lie between each of the tarsal bones and its immediate neighbors, making a very complicated structure. The movement of most of these joints is very small, as there are ligaments crossing the joints, and the joint surfaces are not shaped for large movements. As a result, the midtarsal joints may be considered together to provide a flexible linkage between the hindfoot and the forefoot, which permits a small amount of movement in all directions.

The *tarsometatarsal* joints, between the cuboid and the cuneiforms proximally and the five metatarsals distally, are capable of only small gliding movements because of the relatively flat joint surfaces and the ligaments binding the metatarsals to each other and to the tarsal bones. There are also joint surfaces between adjacent metatarsals, except for the medial one.

The *metatarsophalangeal* and *interphalangeal* joints consist of a convex proximal surface fitting into a shallow concave distal surface. The metatarsophalangeal joints permit abduction and adduction as well as flexion and extension; the interphalangeal joints are restricted by their ligaments

Figure 1.6 Medial side of the right foot. The medial arch consists of the calcaneus, talus, navicular, cuneiforms and medial three metatarsals.

Figure 1.7 Lateral side of the right foot. The lateral arch consists of the calcaneus, cuboid and lateral two metatarsals.

to flexion and extension, the range of flexion being greater than that of extension. In walking, the most important movement in this region is extension at the metatarsophalangeal joints.

No description of the anatomy of the foot is complete without a mention of the arches. The bones of the foot are bound together by ligamentous structures, reinforced by muscle tendons, to make a flexible structure that acts like two strong curved springs, side by side. These are the longitudinal arches of the foot, and they cause the body weight to be transmitted to the ground primarily through the calcaneus posteriorly and the metatarsal heads anteriorly. The midfoot transmits relatively little weight directly to the ground because it is lifted up, particularly on the medial side. The posterior end of both arches is the calcaneus. The *medial arch* (Fig. 1.6) goes upwards through the talus, and then forward and gradually down again through the navicular and cuneiforms to the medial three metatarsals, which form the distal end of the arch. The *lateral arch* (Fig. 1.7) passes forwards from the calcaneus through the cuboid to the lateral two metatarsals.

Muscles and tendons

Muscles are responsible for movements at joints. Most muscles are attached to different bones at their two ends, and cross over one joint (*monarticular*

Figure 1.8 Superficial muscles of the right leg.

muscle), two joints (*biarticular* muscle) or several joints (*polyarticular* muscle). In many cases the attachment to one of the bones covers a broad area, whereas at the other end it narrows into a *tendon*, which is attached to the second bone. It is usual to talk about a muscle as having an origin and an insertion, although these terms are not always clearly defined. Ligaments and tendons are obviously similar and are frequently confused. As a general rule, ligaments connect two bones together whereas tendons connect muscles to bones.

The account that follows gives very brief details of the muscles of the pelvis and lower limb, including their major actions. Most muscles also have secondary actions, which may vary according to the position of the joints, particularly with biarticular muscles. The larger and more superficial muscles are illustrated in Fig. 1.8.

Muscles acting only at the hip joint

1. *Psoas major* originates from the front of the lumbar vertebrae. *Iliacus* originates on the inside of the pelvis. The two tendons combine to form the *iliopsoas*, inserted at the lesser trochanter of the femur; the main action of these two muscles is to flex the hip.
2. *Gluteus maximus* originates from the back of the pelvis and is inserted into the back of the shaft of the femur near its top; it extends the hip.
3. *Gluteus medius* and *gluteus minimus* originate from the side of the pelvis and are inserted into the greater trochanter of the femur; they primarily abduct the hip.
4. *Adductor magnus*, *adductor brevis* and *adductor longus* all originate from the ischium and pubis of the pelvis. They insert in a line down the medial side of the femur and adduct the hip.
5. *Quadratus femoris*, *piriformis*, *obturator internus*, *obturator externus*, *gemellus superior* and *gemellus inferior* originate in the pelvis and insert close to the top of the femur; they all externally rotate the femur, although most also have secondary actions.
6. *Pectineus* originates on the pubis of the pelvis; it runs laterally and inserts on the front of the femur, near the lesser trochanter; it flexes and adducts the hip.

Internal rotation of the femur was not mentioned in the above list; it is achieved as a secondary action by gluteus medius, gluteus minimus, psoas major, iliacus, pectineus and tensor fascia lata (described below).

Muscles acting across the hip and knee joints

1. *Rectus femoris* originates from around the anterior inferior iliac spine of the pelvis and inserts into the quadriceps tendon; it flexes the hip, as well as being part of the *quadriceps* – a group of four muscles that extend the knee.
2. *Tensor fascia lata* originates from the pelvis close to the anterior superior iliac spine and is inserted into the iliotibial tract – a broad band of fibrous tissue which runs down the outside of the thigh and attaches to the head of the fibula. The muscle abducts the hip and the knee.
3. *Sartorius* is a strap-like muscle originating at the anterior superior iliac spine of the pelvis and winding around the front of the thigh to insert on the front of the tibia on its medial side; it is mainly a hip flexor.
4. *Semimembranosus* and *semitendinosus* are two of the *hamstrings*. Both originate at the ischial tuberosity of the pelvis and are inserted into the medial condyle of the tibia; they extend the hip and flex the knee.
5. *Biceps femoris* is the third hamstring; it has two origins – the long head comes from the ischial tuberosity and the short head from the middle of the shaft of the femur. It inserts into the lateral condyle of the tibia and is a hip extensor and knee flexor.
6. *Gracilis* runs down the medial side of the thigh from the pubis to the back of the tibia on its medial side; it adducts the hip and flexes the knee.

Muscles acting only at the knee joint

1. *Vastus medialis*, *vastus intermedius* and *vastus lateralis* are three elements of the quadriceps muscle. They all originate from the upper part of the femur, on the medial, anterior and lateral sides respectively. The fourth element of the quadriceps is rectus femoris, described above. The four muscles combine to become the quadriceps tendon. This surrounds the patella, and continues beyond it as the patellar tendon, which inserts into the tibial tubercle. Quadriceps is the only muscle that extends the knee.
2. *Popliteus* is a small muscle behind the knee; it flexes and helps to unlock the knee by internally rotating the tibia at the beginning of flexion.

Muscles acting across the knee and ankle joints

1. *Gastrocnemius* originates from the back of the medial and lateral condyles of the femur; its tendon joins with that of the soleus (and sometimes also the plantaris) to form the *Achilles tendon*, which inserts into the back of the calcaneus. The main action of these muscles is to plantarflex the ankle, although the gastrocnemius is also a flexor of the knee.
2. *Plantaris* is a very slender muscle running deep to the gastrocnemius from the lateral condyle of the femur to the calcaneus; it is a feeble plantarflexor of the ankle.

Muscles acting across the ankle and subtalar joints

1. *Soleus* arises from the posterior surface of the tibia, fibula and the deep calf muscles. Its tendon joins with that of the gastrocnemius (and sometimes plantaris) to plantarflex the ankle. The soleus and gastrocnemius together are called the *triceps surae*.
2. *Extensor hallucis longus, extensor digitorum longus, tibialis anterior and peroneus tertius* form the anterior tibial group. They originate from the anterior aspect of the tibia and fibula and the interosseous membrane. The former two are inserted into the toes, which they extend; the latter two are inserted into the tarsal bones and raise the midfoot on the medial side (tibialis anterior) or lateral side (peroneus tertius). Tibialis anterior is the main ankle dorsiflexor; the others are weak dorsiflexors.
3. *Flexor hallucis longus, flexor digitorum longus, tibialis posterior, peroneus longus* and *peroneus brevis* are the deep calf muscles, and all arise from the back of the tibia, fibula and interosseous membrane. The former two are flexors of the toes; the peronei are on the lateral side and evert the foot; tibialis posterior is on the medial side and inverts it. All five muscles are weak ankle plantarflexors.

Muscles within the foot

1. *Extensor digitorum brevis* and the *dorsal interossei* are on the dorsum of the foot; the former muscle extends the toes and the latter muscles abduct and flex the toes.

2. *Flexor digitorum brevis*, *abductor hallucis* and *abductor digiti minimi* form the superficial layer of the sole of the foot; they flex the toes and abduct the big toe and the little toe, respectively.
3. *Flexor accessorius*, *flexor hallucis brevis* and *flexor digiti minimi brevis* form an intermediate layer in the sole of the foot; between them they flex all the toes.
4. The *adductor hallucis* is in two parts – the oblique and transverse heads. It adducts the big toe.
5. The *plantar interossei* and the *lumbricals* lie in the deepest layer of the sole of the foot; the former adduct and flex the toes; the latter flex the proximal phalanges and extend the distal ones.

The above five groups of muscles are known together as the *intrinsic muscles* of the foot.

Spinal cord and spinal nerves

The *spinal cord* is an extension of the brain, and plays an active role in the processing of nerve signals. Like the brain itself, it consists of white matter, which is bundles of nerve fibers, and gray matter, which contains many cell bodies and nerve endings, where the synapses (connections) between nerve cells take place. The spinal cord lies within the spinal canal, which is formed in front by the vertebral bodies and behind by the neural arches of the vertebrae (Fig. 1.9). The vertebrae are divided into four groups – cervical (seven vertebrae), thoracic (twelve), lumbar (five) and sacral (five). It is usual to use abbreviated names – for example, the fourth thoracic vertebra is known as T4.

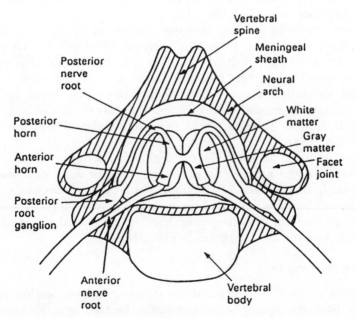

Figure 1.9 Cross-section of vertebra, spinal cord and nerve roots.

Figure 1.10 Spinal cord and spinal nerves, with main functions served.

The spinal cord is shorter than the spinal canal, terminating in adults at approximately the level of the first lumbar vertebra (L1), and a little lower in children. Beyond the end of the spinal cord is a bundle of nerves known as the *cauda equina*, which consists of those nerve roots that enter and leave the lower levels of the spinal canal (Fig. 1.10). There are eight cervical nerve roots but only seven cervical vertebrae; each nerve root except the eighth emerges above the correspondingly numbered vertebra. In the remainder of the spine, the nerve roots emerge below the correspondingly numbered vertebrae.

The organization of the *neurons* (nerve cells) of the spinal cord and the peripheral nerves is extremely complicated. It is possible to give only a brief outline here, although further details will be given in the physiology section later in this chapter. The main neurons responsible for muscle contraction pass down from the brain as *upper motor neurons* in the descending tracts of the spinal cord. At the appropriate spinal level they enter the gray matter and connect with the *lower motor neurons*, also called *efferent* neurons. The axons (nerve fibers) of these cells pass out of the spinal cord through the *anterior root*, combine with other spinal roots and then split into smaller and smaller nerves, finally reaching the muscle itself.

Nerve fibers also pass in the opposite direction, from the muscles, skin and other structures to the spinal cord. They enter the spinal cord at the *posterior root*, having passed through the *posterior root ganglion*, a swelling that contains the cell bodies of the neurons. These *afferent* neurons transmit many different types of sensory information. Some connect with the nerve fibers that pass up the spinal cord to the brain in the ascending tracts, while others synapse with other nerve cells at the same or nearby spinal levels. Connections within the spinal cord are responsible for the spinal reflexes, which will be referred to later.

When the spinal cord is damaged by accident or disease, the outcome depends both on the spinal level at which the damage occurred, and on whether the cord was totally or partially transected (cut through). A wide variety of disabilities may result from incomplete destruction of the spinal cord. If the cord is totally transected the upper motor neurons are unable to control the muscle groups at or below that level, so voluntary control of those muscles is lost. There is also a total loss of sensation below the level of the damage. However, at levels below the damaged area there is usually preservation of the lower motor neurons, the sensory nerves and the spinal reflexes. Injury to the vertebral column below L1 will damage the cauda equina rather than the spinal cord. The cauda equina consists of lower motor neurons and sensory fibers, and damage to it produces a totally different clinical picture from damage to the spinal cord itself.

Patients paralyzed at the level of the cervical spine are *tetraplegic* or *quadriplegic*, with paralysis of the arms and legs. With a cervical lesion above C4 the diaphragm is also paralyzed, making breathing difficult or impossible, and the chances of survival are poor. At the lower cervical levels some arm or hand function is preserved. Where the spinal cord damage is at thoracic or lumbar level only the legs are paralyzed and the patient is *paraplegic*. Where only the cauda equina is damaged the patient has an incomplete paraplegia, and may be able to walk wearing some form of orthosis (an external support, also known as an orthotic, brace or caliper). Patients with paralysis restricted to one side of the body are *hemiplegic*. Sometimes the suffix '-paretic' is used in place of '-plegic'; it implies an incomplete paralysis.

The area of skin served by the sensory nerves from a particular spinal root is known as a *dermatome*. The distribution of the dermatomes for all the spinal nerves is shown in Fig. 1.11. In the legs, the anterior surface is innervated by the higher spinal segments and the posterior by the lower ones; loss of sensation from the buttocks and perineum is likely to follow spinal injury at almost any level.

Peripheral nerves

On emerging from the spinal cord, the spinal roots from adjacent levels form a network known as a *plexus*. The peripheral nerves that emerge from such a plexus usually contain nerve fibers from several adjacent spinal roots. The peripheral nerves supplying the muscles of walking all arise from either the *lumbar plexus* or the *sacral plexus*. Table 1.1 gives brief details of the motor and sensory distribution of the nerves arising from the lumbar plexus, and Table 1.2 the corresponding information for the sacral plexus (sometimes called the lumbosacral plexus).

Figure 1.11 Sensory distribution (dermatomes) of spinal nerve roots.

Physiology

Again, the text that follows is only intended to give an overview of the most important aspects of physiology that apply to gait. There are many good textbooks on the subject; the author uses one by Guyton (1991).

Nerves

Mention has already been made of the nerve cell or *neuron*, the basic element of the nervous system. Although neurons in different parts of the nervous system vary considerably in structure, they all consist of four basic elements (Fig. 1.12) – *dendrites, cell body, axon* and *presynaptic endings*. Nerve impulses are conducted from the dendrites to the cell body, and thence down the axon to the presynaptic endings. These contain very small packages of a chemical known as a *neurotransmitter*, which is released and crosses a small space known as a *synapse*, to stimulate the dendrite of another neuron. Within the brain and spinal cord, dendrites are stimulated to produce a nerve impulse by the axons of other cells, and in turn the nerve impulse sent along the axon stimulates the dendrites of other neurons. The peripheral nerves contain *motor neurons*, whose axons stimulate muscle fibers, and *sensory neurons*, in which the dendrites are stimulated by the sense organs.

Table 1.1 Distribution of nerves arising from the lumbar plexus

Nerve	Origin	Motor	Sensory
Anterior lumbar nerves	L2–L3	Psoas major	—
Iliohypogastric	T12–L1	Abdominal wall	Abdominal wall Lateral buttocks
Ilioinguinal	T12–L1	Abdominal wall	Abdominal wall Upper thigh Genitalia
Genitofemoral	L1–L2	Genitalia	Upper thigh (anterior) Genitalia
Lateral femoral cutaneous	L2–L3	—	Upper thigh (lateral)
Femoral	L2–L4	Iliacus Pectineus Sartorius Rectus femoris Vastus lateralis Vastus intermedius Vastus medialis	Anterior thigh Medial thigh Medial leg Medial foot Hip joint Knee joint
– Saphenous	L2–L4	—	Medial leg Medial foot Knee joint
Obturator	L2–L4	Obturator externus Pectineus Adductor longus Adductor brevis Adductor magnus Gracilis	Medial thigh Hip joint Knee joint

The brain and spinal cord consist of millions of neurons, connected together in a vast and complex network. A single peripheral nerve consists of the axons and dendrites of hundreds or even thousands of individual neurons. The tissues of the brain, spinal cord and peripheral nerves also contain a number of other types of cell known as *neuroglia*, whose functions are either to provide physical support for the neurons or to perform a variety of maintenance functions.

The *upper motor neurons* arise in several different areas of the brain, but most notably in an area known as the motor cortex, and pass down the spinal cord to the appropriate level, crossing over to the other side at some point in the journey. Within the anterior horn of gray matter the upper motor neurons synapse with the lower motor neurons, as well as with a large number of other neurons that take part in the complex system of motor control.

The *lower motor neurons* or efferent neurons arise in the anterior horns of the spinal cord, emerge from the anterior spinal roots and pass down the peripheral nerves to the muscles. The axon usually branches at its distal end, where it synapses with the muscle cells at a number of *motor end plates*. The nerve impulse causes contraction of the muscle, by a process that will be described later.

Table 1.2 Distribution of nerves arising from the sacral plexus

Nerve	Origin	Motor	Sensory
Superior gluteal	L4–S1	Gluteus minimus Gluteus medius Tensor fascia lata	—
Inferior gluteal	L5–S2	Gluteus maximus	—
Nerve to piriformis	S1–S2	Piriformis	—
Nerve to quadratus femoris	L4–S1	Quadratus femoris Inferior gemellus	Hip joint
Nerve to obturator internus	L5–S2	Obturator internus Superior gemellus	—
Perforating cutaneous	S2–S3	—	Medial buttock
Posterior cutaneous	S1–S3	—	Inferior buttock Posterior thigh Upper calf
Sciatic	L4–S3	Biceps femoris Semimembranosus Semitendinosus Adductor magnus	Knee joint
– Tibial	L4–S3	Gastrocnemius Plantaris Soleus Popliteus Tibialis posterior Flexor digitorum longus Flexor hallucis longus	Lower leg (posterior) Posterior foot Lateral foot Knee joint Ankle joint
– – Medial plantar		Adductor hallucis Flexor digitorum brevis Flexor hallucis brevis	Medial foot Distal toes Tarsal joints
– – Lateral plantar		Remaining muscles of foot	Tarsal foot Lateral joints
– – Common peroneal	L4–S2	—	Knee joint
– – Superficial peroneal		Peroneus longus Peroneus brevis	Anterior leg Dorsal foot
– – Deep peroneal		Tibialis anterior Extensor hallucis longus Extensor digitorum brevis Extensor digitorum longus Peroneus tertius	Great toe Second toe Ankle joint Tarsal joints
Pudendal	S2–S4	Perineum	Genitalia

The *sensory nerves* arise in the sense organs of the skin, joints, muscles and other structures. The sense organ itself stimulates the end of the dendrite of the afferent neuron. The dendrite usually commences as a number of branches; these come together and run up the peripheral nerve to enter the posterior root of the spinal cord. The cell body is in the *posterior root ganglion* (Fig. 1.9), and the axon runs from this ganglion into the spinal cord itself, usually terminating in the posterior horn of gray matter, where it synapses with other neurons. As well as the familiar sensations of touch, temperature, pain and vibration, sensory nerves also carry *proprioception* signals, which are used for feedback in the control of

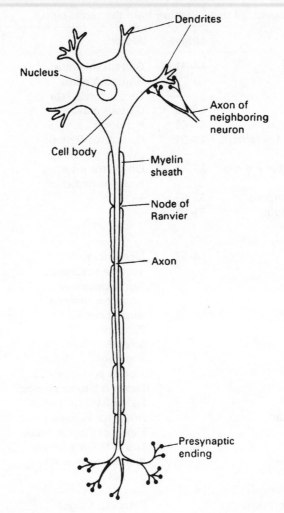

Dendrites

Nucleus

Axon of
neighboring
neuron

Cell body

Myelin
sheath

Node of
Ranvier

Axon

Presynaptic
ending

Figure 1.12 Structure of a neuron.

the limbs. These signals include the positions of the joints and the tension in the muscles and ligaments.

The term *nerve impulse* has been used several times without explanation, and it is now time to rectify this deficiency. The nature of the nerve impulse is a little difficult to grasp, since it is a complicated electrochemical process.

There are different concentrations of ions between the inside of cells (of all types) and the surrounding extracellular fluid. (Ions are atoms or molecules that have gained or lost electrons, making them electrically charged.) The outside layer of a cell is known as the *cell membrane*; it is largely impermeable to sodium ions, and any that leak in are pumped out again. The inside of the cell contains large negatively charged ions, such as proteins, which are unable to pass through the cell membrane. The high concentration of positively charged sodium ions outside the cell and of negative ions inside it causes an automatic compensation, which results in a high concentration of potassium ions on the inside of the cell and of chloride ions outside. The inside of the cell thus has higher concentrations of potassium and large negative ions, while the outside has more sodium and chloride. The result of these imbalances in ionic concentration is a voltage difference between the inside and outside of the cell, across the thickness of the cell membrane. This *membrane potential* can be measured if a suitably small electrode is inserted. The normal resting membrane potential for a neuron is around $-70\,$mV, the negative sign indicating that the inside of the cell is negative with respect to the outside.

All body cells exhibit a membrane potential, but nerve and muscle cells differ from other cells in that they can manipulate it by altering the permeability of the cell membrane to sodium and potassium ions. This is the mechanism by which both nerve impulses and muscular contraction are propagated. If the membrane potential is lowered by about $20\,$mV the membrane suddenly becomes extremely permeable to sodium ions, which enter rapidly from the extracellular fluid. While these ions are entering, the membrane potential is reversed to about $+40\,$mV and it is said to be *depolarized*. The increase in permeability to sodium ions is short lived and is followed by an increased permeability to potassium ions, which leave the cell, thus restoring the ionic balance and returning the membrane potential to $-70\,$mV. The actual number of ions crossing the cell membrane is small and the overall composition of the cell is not affected to any appreciable extent; it is only when the sodium ions have entered, but before the potassium ions have left, that the membrane potential is reversed. The change in membrane potential by around $110\,$mV, from $-70\,$mV to $+40\,$mV, is known as an *action potential*.

Under normal circumstances an action potential in a neuron begins in the synapses, in response to the neurotransmitters released from the presynaptic endings of the axons of other neurons. Some of these are excitatory, which means that they reduce the membrane potential, and some are inhibitory, in that they increase it. This combination of excitatory and inhibitory influences permits the addition and subtraction of nerve impulses. If the net effect of the various excitatory and inhibitory influences causes the membrane potential to fall by around $20\,$mV, an action potential will occur in that region of the neuron. This action potential spreads from its origin, crossing the cell body and running down the axon to its termination.

The action potential is an all-or-none phenomenon, its size and shape being independent of the intensity of the stimulus providing it is above the threshold – there are no larger or smaller action potentials. However, a nerve can pass action potentials either one after another in quick succession, or only occasionally and separated by long intervals. Thus it is the frequency of the nerve impulses, not their size, which carries the information on how hard the muscle is to be contracted, for example, or on the temperature of the skin.

Fig. 1.13 shows an action potential passing along an axon from left to right. At its leading edge, sodium ions enter the axon, producing a region with reversed polarity. At the trailing edge of the action potential, potassium ions leave the axon and the membrane potential is restored. The depolarized region has a membrane potential of $+40\,$mV, whereas the surrounding regions have a membrane potential of around $-70\,$mV.

Figure 1.13 Propagation of an action potential along an axon. Electric current flows from positive regions (+) to negative regions (−).

This is equivalent to a tiny battery producing 110 mV, and an electric current flows between the depolarized region and the surrounding normal regions of cell membrane. The passage of this electric current causes a drop in the membrane potential sufficient to generate an action potential in the normally polarized region in front, enabling the action potential to spread along the nerve. The region immediately behind an action potential becomes *refractory*, meaning that it cannot be stimulated again for a few milliseconds, so the action potential only moves in one direction.

The description so far has ignored the fact that many nerve fibers, particularly those required to send impulses quickly over long distances, are enclosed in a *myelin sheath* (as shown in Fig. 1.12). Myelin is a fatty substance that surrounds nerve fibers, both axons and dendrites, as a series of sleeves, with gaps between them known as *nodes of Ranvier*. Since myelin is an insulator, it prevents the electric current from passing through the cell membrane close to an area of depolarization, forcing it instead to pass through the next node of Ranvier, some distance along the nerve fiber. The effect of this is to cause the action potential to pass down the fiber in a series of jumps, known as *saltatory conduction*, which is much faster than the continuous propagation seen in unmyelinated fibers. A number of neurological diseases, most notably multiple sclerosis, are associated with loss of myelin from nerve fibers, with serious consequences to the functioning of the nervous system.

The speed at which nerve impulses travel depends on two things – the diameter of the nerve fiber, and whether or not it is myelinated. Three speeds of fiber are found within the nervous system, known as types A, B and C. Type A fibers are all myelinated, and are further divided by their conduction velocities into three: alpha (α) – about 100 m/s; beta (β) – about 60 m/s; and gamma (γ) – about 40 m/s. Type B and C fibers are unmyelinated, with conduction velocities around 10 m/s and 2 m/s respectively. The type A fibers are the most important in gait analysis, especially the alpha fibers, which are used for the motor nerves to muscles and the faster sensory nerves such as touch. The gamma fiber is of particular importance in muscle physiology, and will be referred to again later.

When an unmyelinated nerve fiber becomes damaged, recovery of function is usually impossible because of the formation of scar tissue. For this reason, very little recovery of neuronal function takes place following damage to the brain or spinal cord, although function may be partially restored by the use of alternative neurological pathways. Myelinated fibers can recover, providing the cell body remains alive and the myelin sheaths remain in line; the nerve fiber regrows down the sheath at the rate of a few millimeters a week. In practice, if a complete nerve is divided and reconnected most of the nerve fibers will enter the wrong myelin sheaths, although a sufficient number may be correctly connected to provide useful sensory and motor function.

Muscles

The human body contains three types of muscle – smooth, cardiac and skeletal. The description that follows is of *skeletal muscle*, which is responsible for the movement of the limbs. It is also known as voluntary or striated muscle.

A muscle is made up of hundreds of *fascicles* (Fig. 1.14), which in turn consist of hundreds of *muscle fibers*. These large multinucleated cells (cells with many nuclei) are the basic units of muscle tissue. The fiber is itself made up of hundreds of *myofibrils*, which have a characteristic striated (striped) appearance. The striations are due to a regular arrangement of *filaments*, which are made of two types of protein – *actin* and *myosin*. It is the sliding of these filaments past each other, by the formation and destruction of cross-bridges, which is responsible for muscle contraction.

The various light and dark bands in the myofibril are identified by letters. The thin, dark 'Z' line is the origin of the slender actin filaments (Fig. 1.15). These are interleaved with the thicker myosin filaments, which

Figure 1.14 Macroscopic and microscopic structure of muscle.

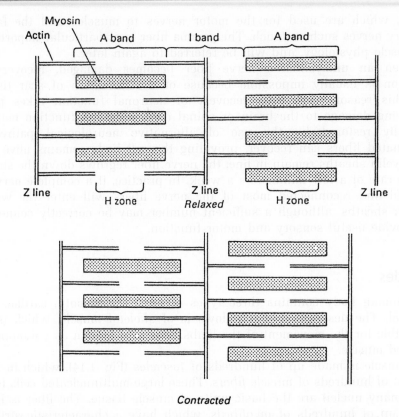

Contracted

Figure 1.15 Sliding of actin and myosin filaments during muscular contraction.

form the 'A' band. The 'I' band and 'H' zone change their width during muscular contraction, as they represent the areas where the actin and myosin, respectively, are *not* overlapped – they were named before the process of contraction was understood!

There is an extremely complicated arrangement of membranes surrounding the myofibrils within the muscle fiber. It is responsible for the transport of nutrients and waste products, and the transmission of the muscle action potential. Outside the muscle fibers are the blood capillaries and the terminal branches of the motor nerves, which connect to the muscle fibers at *motor endplates*, also known as neuromuscular junctions. On average, a single motor nerve will connect to about 150 muscle fibers, the combination of the neuron and the muscle fibers it innervates being known as a *motor unit*.

When an action potential passes down a nerve to the motor endplate, it results in the release of the transmitter substance *acetylcholine (ACH)*. This depolarizes the cell membrane of the muscle fiber, and causes a spreading wave of depolarization. As this *muscle action potential* spreads throughout the muscle fiber, it causes the release of calcium ions, which are the trigger for muscle contraction. Cross-bridges form between the actin and myosin molecules, pulling them together. The tension is maintained for a brief period and then released if no further action potential occurs, the calcium ions being removed by the *calcium pump*. The electrical activity

Figure 1.16 Response of a single muscle fiber to single stimulation, and to repeated stimulation at low and high frequencies.

of muscle action potentials can be detected, and is known as the *electro-myogram (EMG)*.

The energy for muscular contraction comes from the release of a high-energy phosphate group by a chemical known as *adenosine triphosphate (ATP)*. The regeneration of ATP requires the expenditure of metabolic energy, and a failure to keep up with the demand results in muscle fatigue. There are two metabolic pathways involved in regenerating ATP. One uses up chemicals stored within the cell, without the need for oxygen, and is known as *anaerobic*; the other requires oxygen and nutrients to enter the muscle fiber from the bloodstream, and is known as *aerobic*. Anaerobic processes are quickly exhausted, although they can provide brief bursts of powerful contraction. For more sustained muscular effort, aerobic metabolism is required. Following anaerobic respiration a muscle will have an *oxygen debt*, which will need to be repaid by aerobic respiration, to remove lactic acid, which accumulates in the muscle.

If a single nerve impulse stimulates a muscle, it will respond, after a short pause known as the *latent period*, with a brief contraction known as a *twitch* (Fig. 1.16). If the motor nerve delivers a second nerve impulse during the latent period, it has no effect. If the nerve is repeatedly stimulated but there is sufficient time for one twitch to end before the next occurs, the force of contraction will increase over the first few twitches – a phenomenon known as *treppe*. If there is insufficient time for the muscle to relax before it is stimulated again, the force will build up as a *tetanus*. (The disease of the same name results in muscular contraction due to bacterial toxins.) The muscular contractions seen in gait are all tetanic. The force that a muscle is able to generate in a tetanic contraction depends on a number of factors, particularly the strength of stimulation, the cross-sectional area of the muscle, the speed of contraction, and the direction of contraction. The greatest force is usually produced when the muscle length is close to its resting length. If a muscle shortens to its minimum length its force of contraction falls to zero (*active insufficiency*). If the muscle becomes stretched well beyond its resting length it develops tension passively through stretching, but little tension can be developed through active contraction (*passive insufficiency*).

There are a number of different types of muscle fiber, the main subdivision being into types I and II. The type of muscle fiber depends on the type of stimulation reaching it down the motor nerve, and all the fibers in a single motor unit are of the same type. *Type I fibers* are dark in color, they contract and relax slowly, are fatigue-resistant, and are used primarily for the sustained contractions used for posture control. *Type II fibers* are pale in color, fast to contract and relax, and are easily fatigued. They are mainly used for brief bursts of powerful contraction. Depending on their function in the body, different muscles have different proportions of fast and slow fibers. This is also seen in poultry, where the red meat in the leg muscles is used for sustained contraction and the white meat in the wing muscles for bursts of powerful contraction. A change in the stimulation pattern will cause a change in the fiber type in the course of a few weeks, despite the fact that the fiber types differ in the actual structure of the myosin. This ability to alter the fiber type becomes very important when electrical stimulation is used on paralyzed muscles.

When a muscle contracts, not all the motor units are active at the same time. If a stronger contraction is needed, further motor units are brought into use, a process known as *recruitment*.

If a muscle generates tension without changing its length, the contraction is known as *isometric*. If the muscle changes its length but the force of contraction remains the same, the contraction is *isotonic*. One normally thinks of a muscle shortening as it contracts – a *concentric contraction*. However, it is quite usual, particularly in gait, for a muscle to produce tension while it is lengthening – an *eccentric contraction*. For example, the quadriceps undergoes an eccentric contraction as you sit down. The muscle that is responsible for a particular action is known as an *agonist*. If two or more muscles act together, they are known as *synergists*; muscles that oppose agonists are known as *antagonists*. As a general rule, contraction of one set of muscles results in *reciprocal inhibition* of opposing muscles.

Muscle atrophy is the term used to describe the loss of bulk and strength of a muscle when it is not used. If the motor nerve is intact, the muscle fibers will become smaller but their numbers remain the same, and subsequent restoration of muscle stimulation will lead to a full recovery of function. This happens, for example, when a limb is encased in plaster following a fracture. This type of muscle atrophy also occurs in spinal cord injury where the upper motor neurons are destroyed but the lower motor neurons remain intact. In contrast, if the lower motor neuron is destroyed, the muscle fibers shrink and become replaced by fibrous tissue. This leads to an irreversible form of muscle atrophy, such as is seen following poliomyelitis and after damage to the cauda equina or peripheral nerves.

Spinal reflexes

The lower motor neurons receive nerve impulses both from the brain and from other neurons within the spinal cord. The two areas of the brain chiefly concerned with posture and movement are the *motor cortex*, which is responsible for voluntary movement, and the *cerebellum*, which is responsible for generating patterns of muscular activity. The motor cortex and its associated nerves are known as the *pyramidal system*; the cerebellum and some associated brain centers, with their associated nervous pathways, are known as the *extrapyramidal system*. Within the spinal cord itself, the influences of other neurons give rise to the *spinal reflexes*. There are also pattern generators for each limb within the spinal cord, which are capable of producing alternating flexion and extension.

The brain and higher centers exert an inhibitory influence on spinal reflexes, which as a result are often very weak in normal individuals. However, the reflexes may become very strong due to the loss of this inhibition in patients who have suffered damage to the brain or spinal cord.

One of the most important spinal reflexes is the *stretch reflex*, which is responsible for the knee-jerk when the patellar tendon is struck by a small hammer. When a muscle is stretched, *stretch receptors* within it are stimulated, sending nerve impulses to the spinal cord along fast sensory neurons. Within the cord these neurons synapse with and stimulate the lower motor neurons of the same muscle, causing it to contract. The stretch receptors are within the *muscle spindles*, and attached to very small *intra-fusal muscle fibers*, which are innervated by thin, relatively slow *gamma motor neurons*. These adjust the length of the spindle as the main muscle contracts and relaxes, so that it continues to work over the complete range of muscle lengths. The intrafusal fibers are also able to alter the 'sensitivity' of the stretch receptor. The stretch reflex provides a feedback system for maintaining the position of a muscle despite changes in the force applied to it.

The stretch reflex is unusual in that it involves only a single synapse, between the sensory and motor neurons, making it a *monosynaptic reflex*. Most reflexes are *polysynaptic*, involving many intermediate neurons, and often involving neurons on both sides of the spinal cord and at more than one spinal level.

Partly because of the stretch reflex and partly through a continuous low level of activity in the motor neurons, most muscles show a certain amount of resistance to being stretched – this is known as *muscle tone*. In some individuals this effect is exaggerated, giving the clinical condition of *spasticity* in which muscle tone is very high, small movements of the limb being opposed by strong muscular contractions. Spasticity is an important cause of gait abnormalities. It usually results from the loss of some or all of the inhibitory influence of the higher centers on the spinal reflexes, and is often seen in patients with brain damage (as in cerebral palsy) or following damage to the spinal cord. A related phenomenon, also seen in gait, is *clonus*, in which a muscle produces a series of contractions one after the other in response to being stretched.

Many different types of sensory organ in the tissues are responsible for spinal reflexes. Those of particular importance in gait analysis are the muscle spindle, referred to above, and the *Golgi organ*. The latter is a stretch receptor in tendons, which inhibits muscular contraction if the force applied to the tendon, either actively or passively, becomes dangerously large. Pain receptors in the limb may elicit the *flexor withdrawal reflex*, in which the flexor muscles contract and the extensors relax, hopefully to remove the limb from whatever is causing the pain. There is also a *crossed extensor reflex*, where contraction of flexors on one side is accompanied by contraction of extensors on the other. However, this is very weak in humans, even after spinal cord transection.

Motor control

Walking is accomplished through a complex and coordinated pattern of nerve signals sent to the muscles, which in turn move the joints, the limbs and the remainder of the body. The central pattern generator, which produces this pattern of nerve impulses, is not located in a single place, but consists of networks of neurons in various parts of the brain and spinal cord. Much of the research in this area has been done on experimental animals, but there is some evidence that human locomotion is organized in a similar fashion to that in cats, where a rhythm generating system within the spinal cord is controlled by neural input from higher levels in the brain and receives feedback from sensors in the muscles, joints and skin of the legs (Duysens and Van de Crommert, 1998).

Biomechanics

Biomechanics is a scientific discipline that studies biological systems, such as the human body, by the methods of mechanical engineering. Since gait is a mechanical process that is performed by a biological system, it is appropriate to study it in this way. Mechanical engineering is a vast subject, but the descriptions that follow are limited to those aspects most relevant to gait analysis, especially time, mass, force, center of gravity, moments of force, and motion – both linear and angular. The science of biomechanics can be extremely mathematical, but the basic principles are easy to grasp, and the section ends with a worked example to illustrate this. A good text on the scientific basis of movement is Gowitzke and Milner (1988).

Time

The second (s) and the millisecond (ms) are the primary units for time measurement in biomechanics, although it is still fairly common to find walking speed quoted in meters per minute or even miles per hour. When repeated events occur at short intervals of time, it is usual to quote a frequency in hertz (Hz), 1 Hz being one cycle per second. For example, a typical television-based gait analysis system might measure the positions of markers on a patient's limbs at 50 Hz (corresponding to an interval between samples of 20 ms), and sample the ground reaction force and EMG at 500 Hz (2 ms interval between samples). The relationship between sample interval and frequency is given by:

$$\text{Interval (ms)} = 1000/\text{frequency (Hz)}$$

Mass

As we all live in the earth's gravitational field, we normally use the terms mass and weight to mean the same thing. However, there is a clear distinction between them. The *mass* of an object is the amount of matter contained in it, which does not depend on whether any gravity is present, whereas *weight* is the force exerted by gravity on the object.

For example, in an orbiting spacecraft there is no gravity and all objects are weightless, although they still have mass. This means that you are still likely to be injured if someone throws a moon-rock at you inside a space-craft, even though it doesn't 'weigh' anything! We casually talk about measuring our body 'weight' in kilograms or pounds, but this is incorrect in scientific terms; these are units of mass, not of force.

Force

We are all familiar in general terms with the concept of force, but the scientist uses the term in a particular way. Force is a *vector* quantity, which means that it has both magnitude and direction, in contrast to *scalar* quantities, such as temperature, which have only magnitude. The internationally agreed system for scientific measurement is the Système International (SI). The unit of force in this system is the *newton (N)*. The force applied by normal earth gravity to a mass of 1 kg is 9.81 N; 1 newton is the force exerted by gravity on a mass of about 102 g or $3\frac{1}{2}$ ounces. This is easily visualized as being the weight of an average size apple! The earlier imperial and metric units of force were confusing and are best avoided – conversions can be found in Appendix 2. The direction of a force vector may be stated in any convenient manner, for example 20 N downwards, or 140 N at 30° to the x-axis. However, the direction should never be omitted, unless it is obvious.

The whole science of mechanical engineering is based on the three laws of force propounded by Sir Isaac Newton, which may be paraphrased as follows.

Newton's first law: A body will continue in a state of rest, or of uniform motion in a straight line, unless it is acted upon by an external force.

Newton's second law: An external force will cause a body to accelerate in the direction of the force. The acceleration (a) is equal to the size of the force (F) divided by the mass (m) of the object, as in the equation:

$$a = F/m$$

Newton's third law: To every action there is a reaction, which is equal in magnitude and opposite in direction.

Neglecting the strange behavior of atomic and sub-atomic particles, all physical systems simultaneously obey all three of Newton's laws.

It is easy to remember which law is which if you first imagine a brick just floating in space (first law); then someone pushes it, and it accelerates (second law); as it is accelerating, the brick pushes back on whoever or whatever is pushing it (third law).

It is easy to see that a single force acting in one direction can be balanced out by an equal force acting in the opposite direction. A much more common situation, however, is to have a number of forces acting in different directions, which taken together balance each other out. Providing direction is taken into account, it is possible to add and subtract force vectors – as it is with any other vectors such as velocity or acceleration. To understand how this is possible, it is necessary to appreciate the fact that a single force, acting in a single direction, can be exactly equivalent to a number of different forces acting in other directions. Conversely, any

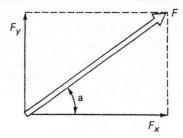

Figure 1.17 Resolution of force *F* into two components at right angles F_x and F_y.

number of separate forces can be represented by an appropriate single force.

The technique used to convert a single force into two forces acting in different directions is known as *resolving into components*. Fig. 1.17 shows how the force *F* can be represented by two smaller forces, F_x and F_y, acting at right angles to each other. The magnitudes of these forces are given by the formulae:

$$F_x = F \times \cos a$$

$$F_y = F \times \sin a$$

where *a* is the angle between *F* and F_x.

The converse process, of combining F_x and F_y to produce *F*, can be performed using these formulae:

$$\text{Magnitude: } F = \sqrt{(F_x{}^2 + F_y{}^2)}$$

$$\text{Angle: } a = \tan^{-1}(F_y/F_x)$$

In order to combine forces they are first resolved into components, using a common system of directions. All the x components are added together, and so are all the y components. The resulting totals are then used to find the single equivalent force. This is illustrated in Fig. 1.18, where two forces, *A* and *B*, are combined to give a resultant force *R*. First, *A* and *B* are resolved into components (A_x, A_y, B_x and B_y). The algebraic sum of the x components gives the x component of the resultant, and similarly with the y components. Since A_x and B_x are in opposite directions, their algebraic sum is actually their difference. The resultant, *R*, is then obtained by recombining the x and y components.

When resolving a force into components it is not necessary that the two components are at right angles, although it makes the calculations much easier because a triangle containing a right angle lends itself to simple geometrical and trigonometrical methods.

Fig. 1.19 shows how graphical methods can be used to combine two forces, *A* and *B*, to give a single resultant force *R*. The two forces are drawn as a scale diagram, with the correct angle between them and the length of the line representing the magnitude of the force. On the left, *A* and *B* are used to draw a parallelogram, the diagonal of which shows the magnitude and direction of *R* – this is the *parallelogram of forces*. On the

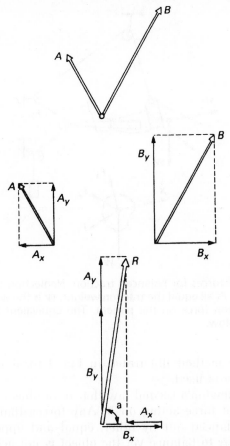

Figure 1.18 Resolution of force A into A_x and A_y, and force B into B_x and B_y. Algebraic addition of A_x and B_x horizontally, and of A_y and B_y vertically, gives the resultant, R.

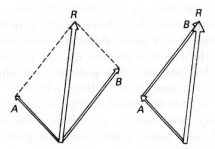

Figure 1.19 Determination of resultant force, R, from forces A and B, by parallelogram of forces (left) and triangle of forces (right).

right, the *triangle of forces* is shown. This does not directly represent the physical arrangement of the forces, since if force A is drawn first, force B is drawn starting at its tip, not its base. The resultant force R is represented by the line that completes the triangle, by joining the base of A to the tip of B. Both the triangle of forces and the parallelogram of forces give the same

Figure 1.20 System of forces for balanced traction. Neglecting friction in the pulleys, F_1, F_2 and F_3 all equal the traction weight. W is the weight of the leg and X the reaction force on the patient. The equivalent free body diagram is shown below.

result, as does the method illustrated in Fig. 1.18; it is a matter of convenience which one is used.

It follows from Newton's second law that if an object is not accelerating, there can be no net force acting on it. Any forces that are acting on the object must be balanced out by other, equal and opposite forces. If the forces do not appear to balance yet the object is not accelerating or decelerating, there must be at least one force that has not been taken into account. This is illustrated in Fig. 1.20, which shows a complicated system of forces in use for the treatment of a fracture of the femur by the old-fashioned method of balanced traction. Such problems are conveniently approached by drawing a *free body diagram* where all the forces are drawn as acting on a shapeless 'lump' floating in space, and in which the sum of all the forces in any given direction must be zero. It can be seen that the forces from the traction system do not balance out; the missing force is the friction that prevents the patient from sliding down the bed (X). It can be found by a graphical method which is an extension of the triangle of forces, or it can be calculated by resolving all the forces into vertical and horizontal components, calculating the 'missing' element of each, and then combining these components to give the magnitude and direction of the missing force.

Center of gravity

Although the mass of any object is distributed throughout every part of it, it is frequently convenient, as far as the effects of an applied force are concerned, to imagine that the whole mass is concentrated at a single point, which is called the *center of gravity (C of G)*. For a regular shape (such as a cube) made of a uniform material, it is easy to see that the center

Figure 1.21 Center of gravity when standing and when bending.

of gravity must be at the geometric center. However, for irregular and changing shapes (such as the human body) it may be necessary to determine it by direct measurement. It is also possible to determine the center of gravity of every part of the body separately, and to find the center of gravity of the whole body by adding these together (by a method which is beyond the scope of this book). It is frequently stated that the center of gravity of the body is just in front of the lumbosacral junction. This is approximately true for a person standing in the anatomical position, but any movement of the body will move the center of gravity. It is not even necessary for the center of gravity to remain within the body – the center of gravity of someone bending down to touch his toes will usually be outside the body, in front of the top of the thigh (Fig. 1.21). An interesting example of this is the technique used by skilled high-jumpers, who curve the body in such a way that although each part of the body in turn passes *over* the bar, the center of gravity actually passes *under* it!

Moment of force

If an adult wishes to play with a small child on a seesaw, he will have to sit much closer to the pivot in order to balance the weight of the child (Fig. 1.22). The action which tends to unbalance the seesaw is the *moment of force*, which is calculated by multiplying the magnitude of the force by its perpendicular distance from the fulcrum or pivot point, this distance commonly being referred to as the *lever arm* or *moment arm*. The

Figure 1.22 The adult on the seesaw will balance the child if the force F_a multiplied by the distance D_a equals the force F_c multiplied by the distance D_c.

moment of force may also be referred to as the torque, the turning moment, or simply the moment. The formula for calculating the moment of force is:

$$M = F \times D$$

where M is the moment of force (in newton-meters, Nm), F is the force (in newtons, N), and D is the distance (in meters, m).

For the system to be in equilibrium, that is for the seesaw to balance, *the sum of the clockwise moments of force must equal the sum of the anti-clockwise moments.* In Fig. 1.22, if the child has a mass of 40 kg she will exert a force due to gravity (F_c) of:

$$40 \text{ kg} \times 9.81 \text{ m/s}^2 = 392.4 \text{ N}$$

If her distance (D_c) from the fulcrum is 4 m, she exerts an anticlockwise moment of:

$$392.4 \text{ N} \times 4 \text{ m} = 1569.6 \text{ Nm}$$

A 70-kg adult will produce a downward force (F_a) of:

$$70 \text{ kg} \times 9.81 \text{ m/s}^2 = 686.7 \text{ N}$$

This will produce an opposing clockwise moment of 1569.6 Nm if he sits at a distance (D_a) from the fulcrum of:

$$1569.6 \text{ Nm}/686.7 \text{ N} = 2.29 \text{ m}$$

The definition of a moment of force refers to the perpendicular distance from the fulcrum. This is very important if opposing moments are produced by forces that act in different directions. Fig. 1.23 illustrates the moments of force about the knee joint when standing with the knee bent. F_1, the weight of the body above this point, is acting at a perpendicular distance a from the point of load bearing. The quadriceps tendon is pulling at an

Figure 1.23 The moment of force due to gravity, F_1 multiplied by a, is opposed by contraction of the quadriceps, producing a moment of force F_2 multiplied by b.

oblique angle relative to the vertical, and the moment of force it provides is the product of the tension in the tendon, F_2, and the perpendicular distance b. It will be noted that the presence of the patella increases the value of b and hence reduces the muscle force needed to produce a given moment of force. For equilibrium, the two moments $(F_1 \times a)$ and $(F_2 \times b)$ must be equal.

The measurement and interpretation of moments of force is essential for the full understanding of normal and pathological gait. Active internal moments are generated by muscular contraction (concentric, isometric or eccentric). Passive internal moments are generated by bone-on-bone forces, and by tension in the soft tissues, especially ligaments. Moments may also be transmitted from adjacent joints. External moments (sometimes referred to as reaction moments) are generally due to gravitational forces. Modern gait analysis systems are able to measure the net moment at the major joints during walking, which is the sum of all the active and passive moments present. Unfortunately, this cannot generally be used to calculate the contraction force of a particular muscle, because there is frequently more than one muscle contracting. An example of this is co-contraction at the hip joint, where flexor and extensor muscles contract at the same time to increase the stability of the joint (Park *et al.*, 1999).

Unfortunately some confusion exists in the literature, because a term like 'flexor moment' is often used without stipulating whether it refers to an internal or external moment. Contraction of a flexor muscle generates an *internal* flexor moment. In contrast, an *external* flexor moment attempts to flex the joint, and is likely to be resisted by the contraction of extensor muscles. To avoid such confusion, it is essential to make it clear whether any moment is internal or external. The gait analysis community now tends to use internal moments, a convention which has been adopted in this book, although the important textbook by Perry (1992) used external moments.

A *couple* is a moment that is produced by two equal forces that are parallel to each other but acting in opposite directions. The forces cancel each other out as far as producing linear motion (displacement or acceleration) is concerned, but work together to produce rotation about a point between them. An example of this is the plantarflexion/knee extension couple, referred to in Chapter 2, which is present in normal walking, and exists in an exaggerated form in some pathological gaits.

In the same way that Newton's third law states that every force is opposed by another equal and opposite force, every moment of force is opposed by an equal and opposite moment. It is impossible to generate a moment unless there is something to 'push back' with an opposing moment. The consequence of this for gait analysis is that if an external force generates a moment at a particular joint (attempting to flex the knee, for example), there *must* be a corresponding internal moment, generated within the joint, to oppose it. In the case of the knee, normally only the quadriceps muscles can provide an internal extensor moment, although generally speaking both muscles and stretched ligaments can generate internal joint moments.

Any object that is supported by the ground will remain stable so long as the *line of gravity* (the line of force passing vertically downwards from the center of gravity) remains within the area on the ground that is supporting it. Should the line of gravity stray outside this area, one of two things can happen – it may automatically correct itself, as happens with a self-righting lifeboat, or it may fall over, as will happen with a pencil balanced on its point. The former is a *stable equilibrium*, where a degree of imbalance produces restoring moments, which push the object back towards the balanced position. The latter is an *unstable equilibrium*, where the moments act to increase the imbalance. When walking at moderate speeds, a further condition exists – a *dynamic equilibrium*, where from instant to instant the equilibrium is unstable, but before there has been time to fall the area of support is moved and equilibrium is restored.

The measurement of the moments generated about the joints of the lower limbs is an important part of scientific gait analysis. Such moments may be expressed in their original units (e.g. newton-meters), or they may be normalized by dividing by body mass, changing the units to newton-meters per kilogram, to make it easier to compare results between individuals of different sizes.

Linear motion

The *velocity* of a moving object is the rate at which its position changes, which usually means the distance it covers in a given time. This is, of course, similar to the everyday concept of speed, except that velocity is a vector and thus has direction as well as magnitude. In measuring gait, the usual unit for velocity is meters per second, which can be abbreviated to either m/s or $m\,s^{-1}$. Sometimes other units are used, such as meters per minute or kilometers per hour, but the SI units are to be preferred.

Acceleration is the rate at which velocity changes; the change may be in either magnitude or direction. An unchanging velocity has an acceleration of zero; a decrease in velocity may be known as negative acceleration, deceleration or retardation. If the velocity is measured in meters per second, the acceleration will be in meters per second per second, abbreviated to m/s² or m s⁻². The acceleration due to gravity has already been mentioned; it has a value of 9.81 m/s².

The relationships between velocity, acceleration and distance traveled are given by four equations:

$$v = u + at$$

$$s = \frac{1}{2}(ut + vt)$$

$$s = ut + \frac{1}{2}at^2$$

$$v^2 - u^2 = 2as$$

where u is the initial velocity (in meters per second, m/s), v is the final velocity (in meters per second, m/s), a is the acceleration (in meters per second per second, m/s²), t is the time (in seconds, s), s is the distance traveled (in meters, m).

The worked example at the end of this chapter uses one of these equations.

Circular motion

An object that is rotating has an *angular velocity*, and if the angular velocity changes there is an *angular acceleration* – such as when a wheel rotating on its axle either speeds up or slows down. In walking, the leg has an angular velocity and undergoes angular acceleration and retardation. Every rotating object has an angular velocity, even if it is not attached to an axle or fulcrum, and a change in that angular velocity is an angular acceleration. In the same way that linear acceleration depends on the presence of a force, angular acceleration will only occur if there is an application of a moment of force.

The detailed mathematics of angular velocity and angular acceleration are beyond the scope of this book, but it is worth saying a few words about the general concepts. Angular velocity is measured as angle turned per unit time, usually as degrees per second or radians per second. Angular acceleration is similarly expressed in degrees (or radians) per second per second. The radian is an obscure unit to non-mathematicians – it is the ratio, within the arc of a circle, of the length of the arc to the radius of the circle. There are 2π radians in a complete circle, giving the relationship:

$$1 \text{ rad} = 180°/\pi = 57.296°$$

When a force applied to an object produces an angular acceleration, the acceleration does not depend solely on the size of the force and the mass of the object, as it does with linear motion. It also depends on the way in which the mass is distributed about the center of gravity – a property known as the *moment of inertia*. An object with the mass concentrated around the outside, such as a flywheel, has a much higher moment of inertia than one with the mass concentrated around the center, such as a cannonball. If a flywheel and a cannonball have the same mass, and are spinning with the same angular velocity, the flywheel will be much more difficult to stop rotating than the cannonball, because of its higher moment of inertia.

Inertia and momentum

The term *inertia* is used to describe the resistance offered by a body to any attempt to set it in motion, or to stop it if it is already moving. It is a descriptive term rather than a measured physical quantity. In the case of linear motion it results from the mass of the object; in the case of rotational motion it results from the moment of inertia.

Momentum exists in two forms – linear and angular. The *linear momentum* (generally just called momentum) of a moving object is calculated by multiplying its velocity by its mass. A force applied to the object will cause it to change its velocity, and hence its momentum. Another way of expressing Newton's second law is to say that the force is equal to the rate of change of momentum. The *angular momentum* of a rotating object is calculated by multiplying its angular velocity by its moment of inertia. A law of conservation of momentum exists, which states that momentum (both linear and angular) cannot be created or destroyed, merely transferred from one object to another.

Momentum has received little attention in gait analysis in the past, but transfers of momentum are involved at a number of key events of the gait cycle, including the heelstrike transient and the end of the swing phase, both of which will be described in more detail in Chapter 2.

Kinetics and kinematics

The terms kinetics and kinematics are commonly used in gait analysis, and they deserve some explanation. *Kinetics* is the study of forces, moments, masses and accelerations, but without any detailed knowledge of the position or orientation of the objects involved. For example, an instrument known as a force platform is used in gait analysis to measure the force below the foot during walking, but it gives no information on the position of the limb or the angle of the joints. *Kinematics* describes motion, but without reference to the forces involved. An example of a kinematic instrument is a camera, which can be used to observe the motion of the trunk and the limbs during walking, but which gives no information on the forces involved. It is obvious that for an adequate quantitative description of an activity such as walking, both kinetic and kinematic data are needed.

Work, energy and power

One of the remarkable features of normal gait is how energy is conserved by means of a number of optimizations. Abnormal gait patterns involve a loss of these optimizations, which may result in excessive fatigue. The measurement, during walking, of energy transfers at individual joints and of overall energy consumption is an important component of scientific gait analysis.

There is a subtle difference in viewpoint between the physical scientist and the biologist as far as work, energy and power are concerned. To the physical scientist, *work* is done when a force moves an object a certain distance. It is calculated as the product of the force and the distance; if a force of 2 N moves an object 3 m, the work done is:

$$2\,N \times 3\,m = 6\,J \text{ (joules)}$$

The *joule* could also be called a newton-meter, but this would cause confusion with the identically named unit used to measure moment of force. *Energy* is the capacity to do work, and is also measured in joules. It exists in two basic forms – *potential* (or stored) energy, and *kinetic* (or movement) energy. In walking there are alternating transfers between potential and kinetic energy, which will be described in Chapter 2. *Power* is the rate at which work is done – a rate of 1 joule per second is a *watt*, which is familiar to users of electrical appliances.

The reason biologists regard these matters slightly differently from physical scientists is that muscles can use energy without shortening – in other words, without doing any physical work. The potential energy stored in the muscles in the form of ATP is converted to mechanical energy in response to the muscle action potential. This energy is still used, even in an eccentric contraction, where the muscle actually gets longer while developing a force, which in physical terms is negative work. In other words, while everyone agrees that walking uphill involves the doing of work, the physicist might expect someone walking downhill to gain energy, whereas in reality the muscles are still activated and metabolic energy is still consumed. Even if a muscle shortens as it contracts, in a concentric contraction, the conversion of metabolic energy to mechanical energy is relatively inefficient, with a typical efficiency of around 25 per cent. The old unit for measuring metabolic energy was the Calorie (the capital C indicating 1000 calories or 1 kilocalorie); the conversion factor is 4200 J or 4.2 kJ equals 1 Calorie (see Appendix 2).

The calculation of the mechanical power generated at joints has become an important part of the biomechanical study of gait. In a rotary movement, when a joint flexes or extends the power (P) is calculated as the product of the moment of force (M) and the angular velocity, omega (ω):

$$P \text{ (watts)} = M \text{ (newton-meters)} \times \omega \text{ (radians per second)}$$

In Chapter 2, reference will be made to the power exchanges across the hip, knee and ankle joints at different stages of the gait cycle. When a muscle is contracting concentrically (e.g. a flexor muscle contracts while a joint is flexing), power is generated. If a muscle contracts eccentrically (e.g. a flexor muscle contracts while a joint is extending), it absorbs power. If a muscle contracts isometrically (e.g. a flexor muscle contracts while the joint angle is unchanging), no power exchange takes place. Although power generation and absorption in the gait cycle is often due to muscle contraction, it is important to realize that the stretching of ligaments and other soft tissues also involves power exchange. If a ligament is stretched it absorbs power, with a resulting storage of potential energy. Some or all of this stored energy may be released later, with a resulting power generation.

In gait analysis it is common practice to divide the joint power by body mass, giving a unit of watts per kilogram, in a similar way to the treatment of joint moments (mentioned above).

Worked example

As an example of the biomechanical principles outlined above, consider the mechanics involved when Wonder Woman (one of the fictional super heroes) jumps from the ground to the top of a building 10 m (32 ft 10 in) high. In order to perform this superhuman feat, she must leave the ground with sufficient velocity to reach the top of the building, despite the deceleration produced by gravity. The distance to be traveled (s) is 10 m, the initial velocity (u) is unknown, the final velocity (v) is zero, and the acceleration (a) is -9.81 m/s^2, which is the acceleration due to gravity – negative because it opposes the movement. The substitution of these values in the equation:

$$v^2 - u^2 = 2as$$

gives the initial velocity (u) as 14.0 m/s.

In order to achieve the necessary velocity, Wonder Woman must accelerate from being stationary in the crouched position to a velocity of 14.0 m/s in the fully stretched position, as her feet leave the ground. The center of gravity of the body, in making this jump, moves through a vertical distance (s) of 0.7 m. The initial velocity (u) is zero, the final velocity (v) is 14.0 m/s. Substituting these values in the equation used above gives the average acceleration (a) as being 140 m/s^2, or about 14 times the acceleration due to gravity, and the duration of the acceleration as 0.1 s.

To achieve this acceleration requires a force acting vertically upwards on the center of gravity. The force is given by the equation:

$$F = m \times a$$

which follows from Newton's second law, where the force (F) is equal to the body mass (m) multiplied by the acceleration (a). If her body mass is 50 kg, the force is: 50 kg $\times$ 140 m/s^2 = 7000 N or 7 kN.

Neglecting the small contribution made by swinging the arms, this force is applied to the center of gravity of the body by extension of the two knees. When the knee is flexed to a right angle, about half way through the acceleration, the center of gravity is about 0.4 m behind the knee joint, whereas the quadriceps tendon is only 0.06 m in front of it. To apply an upward force of 7 kN to the center of gravity, the moment of force required to be generated by each knee is: 7 kN $\times$ 0.4 m/2 = 1.4 kNm.

Since the sum of the clockwise and anticlockwise moments must be equal, each quadriceps must generate a force of: 1.4 kNm/0.06 m = 23.3 kN, or about 48 times body weight. Needless to say, only someone like Wonder Woman can generate quite such large forces in the quadriceps tendon, mere mortals having to settle for about a fifth as much!

The knee extends from about 160° of flexion to 0° in 0.1 s; its angular velocity is thus 1600° per second, or close to 30 radians per second. The power generated is the product of the moment of force and the angular velocity, which for the moment calculated above is: 1.4 kNm $\times$ 30 rad/s = 42 kW. This contrasts with a power generation at the joints in normal walking of 100–300 watts.

References and suggestions for further reading

Anatomy

Palastanga N, Field D, Soames R. (1989) *Anatomy and Human Movement*. Oxford: Heinemann.

Physiology

Duysens J, Van de Crommert HWAA. (1998) Neural control of locomotion; Part 1: the central pattern generator from cats to humans. *Gait and Posture* **7**: 131–141.
Guyton AC. (1991) *Textbook of Medical Physiology*, 8th edn. Philadelphia, PA: W.B. Saunders.

Biomechanics and gait analysis

Gowitzke BA, Milner M. (1988) Scientific bases of human movement, 3rd edn. Baltimore, MD: Williams & Wilkins.
Park S, Krebs DE, Mann W. (1999) Hip muscle co-contraction: evidence from concurrent in vivo pressure measurement and force estimation. *Gait and Posture* **10**: 211–222.
Perry J. (1992) *Gait Analysis: Normal and Pathological Function*. Thorofare, NJ: SLACK Incorporated.

2

Normal gait

In order to understand pathological gait it is necessary first to understand normal gait, since this provides the standard against which the gait of a patient can be judged. However, there are two pitfalls that need to be borne in mind when using this approach. First, the term 'normal' covers both sexes, a wide range of ages, and an even wider range of extremes of body geometry, so that an appropriate 'normal' standard needs to be chosen for the individual who is being studied. If results from an elderly female patient are compared with normal data obtained from physically fit young men there will undoubtedly be large differences, whereas comparison with data from healthy elderly women may show the patient's gait to be well within normal limits appropriate to her sex and age. The second pitfall is that even though a patient's gait differs in some way from normal, it does not follow that this is in any way undesirable, or that efforts should be made to turn it into a 'normal' gait. Many gait abnormalities are a compensation for some problem experienced by the patient, and although abnormal they are nonetheless useful.

Having said all that, it is very important to understand normal gait and the terminology used to describe it before going on to look at pathological gait. This chapter starts with a very brief historical review, then gives an overview of the gait cycle, before going on to study in detail how the different parts of the locomotor system are used in walking.

Walking and gait

As walking is such a familiar activity, it is difficult to define it without sounding pompous. However, it would be remiss not to attempt a definition. Normal human walking and running can be defined as 'a method of locomotion involving the use of the two legs, alternately, to provide both support and propulsion'. In order to exclude running, we must add '... at least one foot being in contact with the ground at all times'. Unfortunately, this definition excludes some forms of pathological gait that are generally regarded as being forms of walking, such as the 'three-point step-through gait' (Fig. 3.21) in which there is an alternate use of two crutches and either one or two legs. It is probably both unreasonable and pointless to attempt a definition of walking which will apply to all cases – at least in a single sentence!

Gait is no easier to define than walking, many dictionaries regarding it as a word primarily for use in connection with horses! This is understandable, since quadruped animals have a repertoire of natural gaits (walking, trotting, cantering, galloping, etc.), as well as some artificial ones such as that taught to 'Tennessee walking horses' in the area where the author lives. Most people, including the author, tend to use the words gait and walking interchangeably. However, there is a difference: the word gait describes 'the manner or style of walking' rather than the walking process itself. It thus makes more sense to talk about a difference in gait between two individuals than a difference in walking.

History

The history of gait analysis has shown a steady progression from early descriptive studies, through increasingly sophisticated methods of measurement, to mathematical analysis and mathematical modeling. Only a brief account of the development of the discipline will be given here. Good reviews of the early years of gait analysis have been given by Garrison (1929), Bresler and Frankel (1950) and Steindler (1953). The more recent history is particularly difficult, as hundreds of papers have been published on the subject in the last two decades. For a fairly complete bibliography, the reader is referred to the CD-ROM *GaitCD*, described in Appendix 3. This section will cite just a few publications that the author thinks are particularly significant.

Descriptive studies

Walking has undoubtedly been observed ever since the time of the first men, but the systematic study of gait appears to date from the Renaissance, when Leonardo da Vinci, Galileo and Newton all gave useful descriptions of walking. The earliest account using a truly scientific approach was in the classic *De Motu Animalum*, published in 1682 by Borelli, who worked in Italy and was a student of Galileo. Borelli measured the center of gravity of the body, and described how balance is maintained in walking by constant forward movement of the supporting area provided by the feet.

The Weber brothers in Germany gave the first clear description of the gait cycle in 1836. They made accurate measurements of the timing of gait and of the pendulum-like swinging of the leg of a cadaver.

Kinematics

Two pioneers of kinematic measurement worked on opposite sides of the Atlantic in the 1870s. Marey, working in Paris, published a study of human limb movements in 1873. He made multiple photographic exposures, on a single plate, of a subject who was dressed in black except for brightly illuminated stripes on the limbs. He also investigated the path of the center of gravity of the body, and the pressure beneath the foot. Eadweard Muybridge (born in England as Edward Muggeridge) became famous in California in 1878 by demonstrating that when a horse is trotting, there are times when it has all four of its feet off the ground at once. The measurements were made using 24 cameras, triggered in quick succession as the horse ran into thin wires stretched across the track. Over the next few years Muybridge made a further series of studies of naked human beings walking, running and performing a surprising variety of other activities!

The most serious application of the science of mechanics to human gait during the nineteenth century was the publication in Germany in 1895 of *Der Gang des Menschen*, by Braune and Fischer. They used a technique similar to Marey's, but using fluorescent strip-lights on the limbs instead of white stripes. The resulting photographs were used to determine the three-dimensional trajectories, velocities and accelerations of the body segments. Knowing the masses and accelerations of the body segments, they were then able to estimate the forces involved at all stages during the walking cycle.

Further valuable work on the dynamics of locomotion was done by Bernstein, working in Moscow in the 1930s. He developed a variety of photographic techniques for kinematic measurement, and studied over 150 subjects. Particular attention was paid to the center of gravity of the individual limb segments and of the body as a whole.

Force platforms

Further progress followed the development of the force platform (also called the forceplate). This instrument has contributed greatly to the scientific study of gait, and is now standard equipment in gait laboratories. It measures the direction and magnitude of the ground reaction force beneath the foot. An early design was described by Amar in 1924, and an improved one by Elftman in 1938. Both were purely mechanical, the force applied to the platform causing the movement of a pointer. In Elftman's design the pointers were photographed by a high-speed cine camera.

Muscle activity

For a full understanding of normal gait, it is necessary to know which muscles are active during the different parts of the gait cycle. The role of the muscles was studied by Scherb in Switzerland during the 1940s, initially by palpating the muscles as his subject walked on a treadmill, then later by the use of electromyography (EMG).

Further advances in the understanding of muscle activity and many other aspects of normal gait were made during the 1940s and 1950s by a very active group working at the University of California at San Francisco and Berkeley, notable among whom was Verne Inman. This group later went on to write *Human Walking* (Inman et al., 1981), which was published just after Inman's death and to many people is the definitive textbook on normal gait. After being out of print for some time, a second edition of the book was published (Rose and Gamble, 1994).

Mechanical analysis

A major contribution to the mechanical analysis of walking was made by Bresler and Frankel (1950), also from the Californian group. They performed free-body calculations for the hip, knee and ankle joints, allowing for ground reaction forces, the effects of gravity on the limb segments, and the inertial forces. The analytical techniques developed by these workers formed the basis of many current methods of modeling and analysis.

An important paper describing the possible mechanisms that the body uses to minimize energy consumption in walking was published by Saunders *et al.* (1953), again from California. Further important work on energy consumption, and in particular the energy transfers between the body segments in walking, was published by Cavagna and Margaria (1966), working in Italy.

By 1960, research began to concentrate on the variability of walking, the development of gait in children, and the deterioration of gait in old age. Patricia Murray, working in Milwaukee, Wisconsin, published a series of papers on these subjects, including a detailed review (Murray, 1967).

Mathematical modeling

Once the motions of the body segments and the actions of the different muscles had been examined and documented, attention passed to the forces generated across the joints. Although limited calculations of this type had been made previously, the study by Paul (1965) was the first detailed analysis of hip joint forces during walking. A subsequent paper by the same author also included an analysis of the forces in the knee (Paul, 1966). Since then there have been many mathematical studies of force generation and transmission across the hip, knee and ankle.

The 1970s and 1980s saw great improvements in methods of measurement. The development of more convenient kinematic systems, based on electronics rather than photography, meant that results could be produced in minutes rather than days. Reliable force platforms with a high frequency response became available, as well as convenient and reliable EMG systems. The availability of high quality three-dimensional data on the kinetics and kinematics of walking and the ease of access to powerful computers made it possible to develop increasingly sophisticated mathematical models. Gait laboratories now routinely measure joint moments and powers for the hip, knee and ankle. Somewhat less reliably, estimates can also be made of muscle, ligament and joint contact forces.

Clinical application

From the earliest days, it has been the hope of most of those working in this field that gait measurements would be found useful in the management of patients with walking disorders. Many of the early workers made studies of people who walked with abnormal gait patterns, and some (notably Amar, Scherb, and the Californian group) attempted to use the results for the benefit of individual patients. However, the results were not particularly impressive.

Since 1960, there has been a more serious attempt to take gait analysis out of the research laboratory and into the clinic. With the improvements in measurement and analytical techniques, the major limitation now is not the ability to produce high quality data, but knowing how best to use these data for the benefit of patients. It is fair to say that in the early days far more progress was made in scientific gait analysis, particularly as applied to normal subjects, than in the application of these techniques for the benefit of those with gait disorders. However, since about 1980 there has been a steady increase in the effective use of gait analysis in the clinical management of patients.

As well as a gradual increase in the clinical use of scientific gait analysis, there has also been a growing interest in the use of observational or visual gait analysis. This has become much easier to perform since video cameras and videocassette recorders (VCRs) have become widely available.

Terminology used in gait analysis

The *gait cycle* is defined as the time interval between two successive occurrences of one of the repetitive events of walking. Although any event could be chosen to define the gait cycle, it is generally convenient to use the instant at which one foot contacts the ground ('initial contact'). If it is decided to start with initial contact of the right foot, as shown in Fig. 2.1, then the cycle will continue until the right foot contacts the ground again. The left foot, of course, goes through exactly the same series of events as the right, but displaced in time by half a cycle.

The following terms are used to identify major events during the gait cycle:

1. Initial contact
2. Opposite toe off
3. Heel rise
4. Opposite initial contact
5. Toe off
6. Feet adjacent
7. Tibia vertical

then back to 1. Initial contact.

These seven events subdivide the gait cycle into seven periods, four of which occur in the stance phase, when the foot is on the ground, and three in the swing phase, when the foot is moving forward through the air (Fig. 2.1). The stance phase, which is also called the support phase or contact phase, lasts from initial contact to toe off. It is subdivided into:

1. Loading response
2. Mid-stance

Figure 2.1 Positions of the legs during a single gait cycle by the right leg (shaded).

3. Terminal stance
4. Pre-swing.

The swing phase lasts from toe off to the next initial contact. It is sub-divided into:

1. Initial swing
2. Mid-swing
3. Terminal swing.

The duration of a complete gait cycle is known as the *cycle time*, which is divided into *stance time* and *swing time*.

Unfortunately, the nomenclature used to describe the gait cycle varies considerably from one publication to another. The present text uses terms that will be understood by most people working in the field; alternative terminology will be given where appropriate. Wall *et al.* (1987) pointed out that the usual terminology is inadequate to describe some severely patho-logical gaits.

Gait cycle timing

Fig. 2.2 shows the timings of initial contact and toe off for both feet during a little more than one gait cycle. Right initial contact occurs while the left foot is still on the ground, and there is a period of *double support* (also

Figure 2.2 Timing of single and double support during a little more than one gait cycle, starting with right initial contact.

known as double limb stance) between initial contact on the right and toe off on the left. During the swing phase on the left side, only the right foot is on the ground, giving a period of *right single support* (or single limb stance), which ends with initial contact by the left foot. There is then another period of double support, until toe off on the right side. *Left single support* corresponds to the right swing phase, and the cycle ends with the next initial contact on the right.

In each double support phase one foot is forward, having just landed on the ground, and the other one is backward, being just about to leave the ground. When it is necessary to distinguish between the two legs in the double support phase, the leg in front is usually known as the leading leg and the leg behind as the trailing leg. The leading leg is in loading response, sometimes referred to as braking double support, initial double support or weight acceptance. The trailing leg is in pre-swing, also known as second, terminal or thrusting double support, or weight release.

In each gait cycle there are thus two periods of double support and two periods of single support. The stance phase usually lasts about 60 per cent of the cycle, the swing phase about 40 per cent, and each period of double support about 10 per cent. However, this varies with the speed of walking, the swing phase becoming proportionately longer and the stance phase and double support phases shorter as the speed increases (Murray, 1967). The final disappearance of the double support phase marks the transition from walking to running. Between successive steps in running there is a *flight phase*, also known as the float, double-float or non-support phase, when neither foot is on the ground. A detailed study of gait cycle timing was published by Blanc *et al.* in 1999.

Foot placement

The terms used to describe the placement of the feet on the ground are shown in Fig. 2.3. The *stride length* is the distance between two successive

Figure 2.3 Terms used to describe foot placement on the ground.

placements of the same foot. It consists of two *step lengths*, left and right, each of which is the distance by which the named foot moves forward in front of the other one. In pathological gait, it is common for the two step lengths to be different. If the left foot is moved forward to take a step and the right one is brought up beside it rather than in front of it, the right step length will be zero. It is even possible for the step length on one side to be negative, if that foot never catches up with the other one. However, the *stride* length, measured between successive positions of the left foot, must always be the same as the stride length measured between successive positions of the right foot, unless the subject is walking around a curve.

This definition of a stride, consisting of one step by each foot, breaks down in some pathological gaits in which one foot makes a series of 'hopping' movements while the other is in the air (Wall et al., 1987). There is no satisfactory nomenclature to deal with this situation.

The *walking base* (also known as the stride width or base of support) is the side-to-side distance between the line of the two feet, usually measured at the mid-point of the back of the heel, but sometimes below the center of the ankle joint. The preferred units for stride length and step length are meters, and for the walking base millimeters.

The *toe out* (or, less commonly, *toe in*) is the angle in degrees between the direction of progression and a reference line on the sole of the foot. The reference line varies from one study to another; it may be defined anatomically, but is commonly the midline of the foot as judged by eye.

It is common experience that you need to walk more carefully on ice than on asphalt. Whether or not the foot slips during walking depends on two things: the coefficient of friction between the foot and the ground, and the relationship between the vertical force and the forces parallel to the walking surface (front-to-back and side-to-side). In normal walking, a co-efficient of friction of 0.35–0.40 is generally sufficient to prevent slippage.

Cadence, cycle time and speed

The *cadence* is the number of steps taken in a given time, the usual units being steps per minute. In most other types of scientific measurement complete cycles are counted, but, as there are two steps in a single gait cycle, the cadence is a measure of half-cycles. Measurement in steps per minute does not conform with the Systéme International (SI). A scientifically acceptable alternative would be to measure cadence in steps per second, but there is currently a trend to replace cadence entirely by a quantity that is inversely related to it – the *cycle time*, also known as the stride time, in seconds:

$$\text{Cycle time (s)} = 120/\text{cadence (steps/min)}$$

The normal ranges for both cadence and cycle time in both sexes at different ages are given in Appendix 1.

The *speed* of walking is the distance covered by the whole body in a given time, and should be measured in meters per second. Many authors use the term 'velocity' in place of 'speed', but this is an incorrect usage of the term, unless the direction of walking is also stated. The instantaneous speed varies from one instant to another during the walking cycle, but the average speed is the product of the cadence and the stride length, providing appropriate units are used. The cadence, in steps per minute, corresponds to half-strides per 60 seconds, or full strides per 120 seconds. The speed can thus be calculated from cadence and stride length using the formula:

$$\text{Speed (m/s)} = \text{stride length (m)} \times \text{cadence (steps/min)}/120$$

If cycle time is used in place of cadence, the calculation becomes much more straightforward:

$$\text{Speed (m/s)} = \text{stride length (m)}/\text{cycle time (s)}$$

The walking speed thus depends on the two step lengths, which in turn depend to a large extent on the duration of the swing phase on each side. The step length is the amount by which the foot can be moved forwards during the swing phase, so that a short swing phase on one side will generally reduce the step length on the other side. If the foot catches on the ground, this may terminate the swing phase and thereby reduce both step length and walking speed.

When making comparisons between individuals, particularly with children, it is sometimes useful to allow for differences in size. This is done by dividing a measurement by some aspect of body size, such as height (stature) or leg length, a procedure generally known as normalization. It is thus fairly common to see walking speed expressed in 'statures per second', or to see measures such as 'step factor', which is step length divided by leg length (Sutherland, 1997).

Since walking speed depends on both cadence and stride length, it follows that speed may be changed by altering only one of these variables, for instance by increasing the cadence while keeping the stride length constant. In practice, however, people normally change their walking speed by adjusting both cadence and stride length. Sekiya and Nagasaki (1998) defined the walk ratio as step length (m) divided by step rate (steps/min), and found that it was fairly constant in both males and females over a range of walking speeds from very slow to very fast. Macellari *et al.*

(1999) performed a detailed study of the relationships between gender, body size, walking speed, gait timing and foot placement.

Outline of the gait cycle

The purpose of this section is to provide the reader with an overview of the gait cycle, to make the detailed description that follows a little easier to follow. The cycle is illustrated by Figs 2.4–2.8 and 2.10–2.20, all of which are taken from a single walk by a 22-year-old normal female, weight 540 N (55 kgf, 121 lbf), walking barefoot with a cycle time of 0.88 s (cadence 136 steps/min), a stride length of 1.50 m and a speed of 1.70 m/s. The individual measurements from this subject do not always correspond to 'average' values because of the normal variability between individuals, although they are all close to the normal range. The measurements were all made in the plane of progression, which is a vertical plane aligned to the direction of the walk; in normal walking it closely corresponds to the sagittal plane of the body. The data were obtained using a Vicon television/computer system and a Bertec force platform. It should be noted that different laboratories use different methods of measurement, so that other publications may quote different values for some of the measured variables. The reader should thus concentrate on the changes in the variables during the gait cycle, rather than on their absolute values.

Some gait studies are performed barefoot, and some with the subject wearing shoes. Oeffinger *et al.* (1999) found small differences in some of the gait parameters between these two conditions in children, but did not consider them to be clinically significant. It is usually at the discretion of the investigator whether or not shoes are worn, although in some cases (e.g. when an orthosis is worn within the shoe) this may be dictated by the subject's condition.

During gait, important movements occur in all three planes – sagittal, frontal and transverse. However, this introductory text will concentrate on the sagittal plane, in which the largest movements occur. For information on the motion in other planes, the reader is referred to more detailed texts such as Inman *et al.* (1981), Perry (1992) or Rose and Gamble (1994).

Fig. 2.4 shows the successive positions of the right leg at 40 ms intervals, measured over a single gait cycle. Fig. 2.5 shows the corresponding sagittal plane angles at the hip, knee and ankle joints. Fig. 2.6 shows the joint moments (in newton-meters per kilogram body mass) and Fig. 2.7 the joint powers (in watts per kilogram body mass). Different authors have used different units for the measurement of moments and powers; those used here are scaled for body mass, but not for the length of the limb segments. In Fig. 2.7, the annotations H1–H3, K1–K4 and A1–A2 refer to the peaks of power absorption and generation described by Winter (1991).

Fig. 2.8 shows a 'butterfly diagram', described by Pedotti (1977) and made up of successive representations, at 10 ms intervals, of the magnitude, direction and point of application of the ground reaction force vector. The vectors move across the diagram from left to right.

Fig. 2.9 gives the typical activity of a number of key muscles or muscle

Figure 2.4 Position of the right leg in the sagittal plane at 40 ms intervals during a single gait cycle.

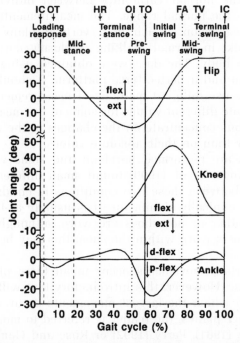

Figure 2.5 Sagittal plane joint angles (degrees) during a single gait cycle of right hip (flexion positive), knee (flexion positive) and ankle (dorsiflexion positive). IC = initial contact; OT = opposite toe off; HR = heel rise; OI = opposite initial contact; TO = toe off; FA = feet adjacent; TV = tibia vertical.

groups during the gait cycle. It is based largely on data from Inman *et al.* (1981), Perry (1992), and Rose and Gamble (1994). Similar though not identical data for these and other muscles were given by Sutherland (1984) and Winter (1991). Although Fig. 2.9 shows a typical pattern, it is not the only possible one. One of the interesting things about gait is the way in which the same movement may be achieved in a number of different ways, and this particularly applies to the use of muscles, so that two people may walk with the same 'normal' gait pattern but using different combinations of muscles. The pattern of muscle usage varies not only from

Figure 2.6 Sagittal plane internal joint moments (newton-meters per kilogram body mass) during a single gait cycle of right hip (extensor moment positive), knee (extensor moment positive), and ankle (plantarflexor moment positive). Abbreviations as in Fig. 2.5.

Figure 2.7 Sagittal plane joint powers (watts per kilogram body mass) during a single gait cycle of right hip, knee and ankle. Power generation is positive, absorption is negative. See text for meaning of H1, H2, etc. Other abbreviations as in Fig. 2.5.

Figure 2.8 'Butterfly diagram' representation of ground reaction force vector at 10 ms intervals. Progression is from left to right.

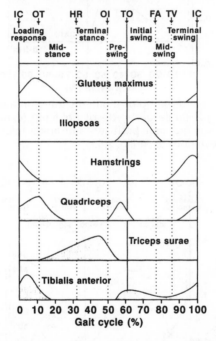

Figure 2.9 Typical activity of major muscle groups during the gait cycle. Abbreviations as in Fig. 2.5. The timings of the events of the gait cycle are typical, and are not derived from a single subject.

one subject to another, but also with fatigue and with walking speed in a single person. The muscular system is said to possess 'redundancy', which means that if a particular muscle cannot be used its functions may be taken over by another muscle or group of muscles. A good review of muscle activity in gait was provided by Shiavi (1985).

Figs 2.10–2.18 show the positions of the two legs and the ground reaction force vector beneath the right foot (where present) at the seven major events of the gait cycle and at two additional points – near the beginning of the loading response (Fig. 2.11) and half way through mid-stance (Fig. 2.13). The description is based on a gait cycle from right initial contact to the next right initial contact. However, the gait cycle could just as well have been defined using the left leg.

Throughout the text, references will be made to the position of the ground reaction force vector relative to the axis of a joint, and to the resulting joint moments. This approach, known as vector projection, is an approximation at best, since it neglects the mass of the leg below the joint in question (especially important at the hip) and also ignores the acceleration and deceleration of the limb segments (which primarily lead to errors in the swing phase). However, the author has used this approach since it makes it much easier to understand joint moments. The graphs for joint moments (Fig. 2.6) and joint powers (Fig. 2.7) were calculated 'correctly', using a method known as inverse dynamics. Wells (1981) discussed the relative merits of these two methods for estimating joint moments.

Upper body: The upper body moves forwards throughout the gait cycle. Its speed varies a little, being fastest during the double support phases and slowest in the middle of the stance and swing phases. The trunk twists about a vertical axis, the shoulder girdle rotating in the opposite direction to the pelvis. The arms swing out of phase with the legs, so that as the left leg and the left side of the pelvis move forwards, so do the right arm and the right side of the shoulder girdle. Murray (1967) found average total excursions of 7° for the shoulder girdle and 12° for the pelvis in adult males walking at free speed. The fluidity and efficiency of walking depend to some extent on the motions of the trunk and arms, but these movements are commonly ignored in clinical gait analysis and have been relatively neglected in gait research. The whole trunk rises and falls twice during the cycle, through a total range of about 46 mm (Perry, 1992), being lowest during double support and highest in the middle of the stance and swing phases. An approximation to this vertical motion can be seen in the position of the hip joint in Fig. 2.4. The trunk also moves from side to side once in each cycle, the trunk being over each leg during its stance phase, as might be expected from the need for support. The total range of side-to-side movement is also about 46 mm (Perry, 1992). The pelvis, as well as twisting about a vertical axis, also tips slightly both backwards and forwards (with an associated change in lumbar lordosis) and from side to side. The spinal muscles are selectively activated so that the head moves less than the pelvis, which is important for providing a stable platform for vision (Prince *et al.*, 1994).

Hip: The hip flexes and extends once during the cycle (Fig. 2.5). The limit of flexion is reached around the middle of the swing phase, and the hip is then kept flexed until initial contact. The peak extension is reached before the end of the stance phase, after which the hip begins to flex again.

Knee: The knee shows two flexion and two extension peaks during each gait cycle. It is more or less fully extended before initial contact, flexes during the loading response and the early part of mid-stance (stance phase knee flexion), extends again during the later part of mid-stance, then starts flexing again, reaching a peak during initial swing (swing phase knee flexion). It extends again prior to the next initial contact.

Ankle and foot: The ankle is usually within a few degrees of the neutral position for dorsiflexion/plantarflexion at the time of initial contact. After initial contact the ankle plantarflexes, bringing the forefoot down onto the ground. During mid-stance the tibia moves forward over the foot and the ankle joint becomes dorsiflexed. Before opposite initial contact the ankle angle again changes, a major plantarflexion taking place until just after toe off. During the swing phase the ankle moves back into dorsiflexion until the forefoot has cleared the ground (around feet adjacent), after which something close to the neutral position is maintained until the next initial contact. In the frontal plane, the heel is slightly inverted (adducted or varus) at initial contact and the forefoot is slightly supinated. The forefoot pronates as it contacts the ground, then moves back into supination as the ankle angle changes from plantarflexion to dorsiflexion, this supinated attitude being maintained as the heel rises and the ankle plantarflexes prior to toe off. Some degree of supination is retained throughout the swing phase.

The gait cycle in detail

Each of the following sections begins with some general remarks about the events surrounding a particular event in the gait cycle, and then describes what is happening in the upper body, hips, knees, ankles and feet, with particular reference to the activity of the muscles. These sections are very detailed, and may be too much to comprehend in one 'pass'. It is suggested that the reader should skip the moments and powers on the first reading, but should go back to them later to gain a deeper understanding of the mechanical processes underlying the gait cycle.

More detailed descriptions of the events of normal gait are given by Murray (1967), Inman *et al.* (1981), Perry (1992), and Rose and Gamble (1994).

Initial contact (Fig. 2.10)

1. *General*: Initial contact is the beginning of the loading response, which is the first period of the stance phase. Initial contact is frequently called heelstrike, since in normal individuals there is often a distinct impact between the heel and the ground, known as the heelstrike transient. Other names for this event are heel contact, footstrike or foot contact. The direction of the ground reaction force changes from generally upwards during the heelstrike transient (Fig. 2.10), to upwards and backwards immediately afterwards, in the loading response (Fig. 2.11). This change in direction can also be seen in the butterfly diagram (Fig. 2.8), where the force vector changes direction immediately after initial contact.

2. *Upper body*: The trunk is about half a stride length behind the leading (right) foot at the time of initial contact. In the side-to-side direction, the trunk is crossing the midline in its range of travel, moving towards the right, as the foot on that side makes contact. The trunk is twisted, the left shoulder and the right side of the pelvis each being at their furthest forwards, and the left arm at its most advanced. The amount of arm swinging varies greatly from one person to another, and it also increases

Figure 2.10 Initial contact position of right leg (solid line), left leg (dashed line) and ground reaction force vector during the heelstrike transient. This illustration also applies to terminal foot contact.

with the speed of walking. At the time of initial contact, Murray (1967) found the mean elbow flexion was 8° and the shoulder flexion 45°.

3. *Hip:* The attitude of the legs at the time of initial contact is shown in Fig. 2.10. The maximum flexion of the hip (generally around 30°) is reached around the middle of the swing phase, after which it changes little until initial contact. The hamstrings are active during the latter part of the swing phase (since they act to prevent knee hyperextension) and gluteus maximus begins to contract around the time of initial contact; together these muscles start the extension of the hip, which will be complete around the time of opposite initial contact (Fig. 2.5).

4. *Knee:* The knee extends rapidly at the end of the swing phase, becoming more or less straight just before initial contact, and then starting to flex again (Figs 2.5 and 2.10). This extension is generally thought to be passive, although Perry (1992) states that it involves quadriceps contraction. Except in very slow walking, the hamstrings contract eccentrically at the end of the swing phase, to act as a braking mechanism to prevent knee hyperextension. This contraction continues into the beginning of the stance phase.

5. *Ankle and foot:* The ankle is generally close to its neutral position in plantarflexion/dorsiflexion at the time of initial contact. This position is usually referred to as 0°, although the angle between the foot and the tibia is actually around 90°. Since the tibia is sloping backwards, the foot slopes upwards and only the heel contacts the ground (Fig. 2.10). The heel is usually slightly inverted (adducted or varus) and the forefoot slightly supinated at this time, and most people show a wear pattern on the lateral side of the heel of the shoe. Tibialis anterior is active throughout swing and in early stance, having maintained dorsiflexion

during the swing phase, and in preparation for the controlled movement into plantarflexion, which occurs following initial contact.

6. *Moments and powers*: At the time of initial contact there is an internal extensor moment at the hip (Fig. 2.6) produced by contraction of the hip extensors, gluteus maximus and the hamstrings (Fig. 2.9). As the hip joint moves in the direction of extension, these muscles contract concentrically and generate power (H1 in Fig. 2.7). The knee shows an internal flexor moment due to contraction of the hamstrings (Fig. 2.9) as they prevent hyperextension at the end of the swing phase. As the knee starts to flex, concentric contraction of the hamstrings, as well as the release of energy stored in the ligaments of the extended knee, results in a short-lived power generation (unnamed peak in Fig. 2.7). Little moment or power exchange occurs at the ankle until just after initial contact.

Loading response (Fig. 2.11)

1. *General*: The loading response is the double support period between initial contact and opposite toe off. During this period, the foot is lowered to the ground by plantarflexion of the ankle. The ground reaction force increases rapidly in magnitude, its direction being upwards and backwards. In the subject used for illustration, loading response occupied the period from 0–7 per cent of the cycle; this is unusually short, loading response typically occupying the first 10–12 per cent of the cycle. Fig. 2.11 represents 2 per cent of the cycle, indicated by a dashed line during loading response in Figs 2.5–2.7.
2. *Upper body*: During loading response the trunk is at its lowest vertical position, about 20 mm below its average level for the whole cycle; its

Figure 2.11 Loading response position of right leg (solid line), left leg (dashed line) and ground reaction force vector 20 ms after initial contact.

instantaneous forward speed is at its greatest, around 10 per cent higher than the average speed for the whole cycle. It continues to move laterally towards the right foot. The arms, having reached their maximum forward (left) and backward (right) positions, begin to return.

3. *Hip:* During loading response the hip begins to extend (Fig. 2.5) through concentric contraction of the hip extensors, gluteus maximus and the hamstrings (Fig. 2.9).

4. *Knee:* From its nearly fully extended position at initial contact, the knee flexes during loading response (Fig. 2.5), initiating the 'stance phase flexion'. This is accompanied by eccentric contraction of the quadriceps (Fig. 2.9) to limit the speed and magnitude of flexion.

5. *Ankle and foot:* The loading response period of the gait cycle, also called the initial rocker, heel rocker or heel pivot, involves plantarflexion at the ankle (Fig. 2.5). The plantarflexion is permitted by eccentric contraction of the tibialis anterior muscle. The movement into plantarflexion is accompanied by pronation of the forefoot and internal rotation of the tibia, there being an automatic coupling between pronation/supination of the forefoot and internal/external rotation of the tibia (Inman *et al.*, 1981; Rose and Gamble, 1994). The direction of the force vector changes from that shown in Fig. 2.10 to that shown in Fig. 2.11 within 10–20 ms.

6. *Moments and powers:* As described above (Initial contact, section 6), the hip shows an internal extensor moment with power generation during the loading response, and the knee shows an internal flexor moment with power generation. At the ankle, the posterior placement of the force vector (Fig. 2.11) produces an external plantarflexor moment. In the normal individual this is resisted by an internal dorsiflexor moment (Fig. 2.6) produced by tibialis anterior (Fig. 2.9), which contracts eccentrically, absorbing power (Fig. 2.7) and permitting the foot to be lowered gently to the ground. Should tibialis anterior fail to generate sufficient moment, the foot dorsiflexes too rapidly, producing an audible 'foot slap'.

Opposite toe off (Fig. 2.12)

1. *General:* Opposite toe off, also known as opposite foot off, is the end of the double support period known as loading response, and the beginning of mid-stance, the first period of single support. The forefoot, which was being lowered by plantarflexion of the ankle, contacts the ground at 'foot flat' (also known as forefoot contact), which generally occurs around the time of opposite toe off. On the opposite (left) side, it marks the end of the stance phase and the beginning of the swing phase. In the subject used for illustration, opposite toe off (Fig. 2.12) occurred at 7 per cent of the cycle and foot flat at 8 per cent of the cycle.

2. *Upper body:* At opposite toe off, the left shoulder and arms, having reached their most advanced position, are now moving back again. Similarly, the pelvis on the right side now starts to twist back towards the neutral position. The trunk, having reached its lowest position during loading response, now begins to gain height but to lose forward speed as a result of the backward and upward direction

Figure 2.12 Opposite toe off position of right leg (solid line), left leg (dashed line) and ground reaction force vector.

of the ground reaction force acting on the center of gravity of the body. This represents a conversion of kinetic energy to potential energy, similar to that seen in a child's swing.

3. *Hip*: The hip flexion angle is around 25° at the time of opposite toe off (Fig. 2.5). The hip continues to extend, by concentric contraction of the gluteus maximus and hamstrings.

4. *Knee*: At opposite toe off the knee is continuing to flex, reaching the peak of stance phase flexion early in mid-stance, after which it begins to extend again (Fig. 2.5). The magnitude of the stance phase flexion is very sensitive to walking speed; it disappears in a very slow walk. Quadriceps contraction (eccentric then concentric) permits the knee to act like a spring, preventing the vertical force from building up too rapidly (Perry, 1974).

5. *Ankle and foot*: As soon as the foot is flat on the ground, around opposite toe off, the direction of ankle motion changes from plantarflexion to dorsiflexion as the tibia moves over the now stationary foot (Fig. 2.5). Both forefoot pronation and internal tibial rotation reach a peak around opposite toe off, and begin to reverse. These two motions are coupled, i.e. they always occur together, due in part to the geometry of the ankle and subtalar joints (Inman et al., 1981; Rose and Gamble, 1994). Tibialis anterior ceases to contract, to be replaced by contraction of the triceps surae (Fig. 2.9).

6. *Moments and powers*: At opposite toe off, the hip continues to have an internal extensor moment with power generation as described above (Initial contact, section 6). At the knee, the force vector lies behind the joint (Fig. 2.12), producing an external flexor moment. This is opposed by an internal extensor moment (Fig. 2.6) generated by the quadriceps muscles (Fig. 2.9). These contract eccentrically, absorbing power (K1 in Fig. 2.7). The line of the ground reaction force begins to move forwards along the foot (Fig. 2.12), causing the internal dorsiflexor moment at the

Figure 2.13 Mid-stance position of right leg (solid line), left leg (dashed line) and ground reaction force vector 100 ms after opposite toe off.

ankle to become smaller, and then to reverse to a plantarflexor moment (Fig. 2.6). Little power exchange occurs at the ankle at this time.

Mid-stance (Fig. 2.13)

1. *General*: Mid-stance is the period of the gait cycle between opposite toe off and heel rise, although the term has been used in the past to describe an event of the gait cycle – the time at which the swing phase leg passes the stance phase leg, corresponding to the swing phase event of feet adjacent. In the subject used for illustration, mid-stance occupied the period from 7 per cent to 32 per cent of the cycle; Fig. 2.13 represents 18 per cent of the cycle, indicated by the dashed line during mid-stance in Figs 2.5–2.7.
2. *Upper body*: The period of mid-stance sees the trunk climbing to its highest point, about 20 mm above the mean level, and slowing its forward speed as the kinetic energy of forward motion is converted to the potential energy of height. The side-to-side motion of the trunk also reaches its peak during mid-stance, the trunk being displaced about 20 mm from its central position towards the side of the stance (right) leg. Like the feet, the arms pass each other during mid-stance, as each follows the motion of the opposite leg. The twisting of the trunk has now disappeared, as both the shoulder girdle and pelvis pass through neutral before twisting the other way.
3. *Hip*: During the mid-stance period the hip continues to extend, moving from a flexed attitude to an extended one (Fig. 2.5). Concentric contraction of gluteus maximus and the hamstrings ceases during this period, as hip extension is achieved by inertia and gravity. Throughout mid-stance and terminal stance, significant muscle activity about the hip joint takes place in the frontal plane. As soon as the opposite foot

has left the ground, the pelvis is supported only by the stance phase hip. Although dipping down slightly on the side of the swinging leg its position is maintained by contraction of the hip abductors, especially gluteus medius and tensor fascia lata.

4. *Knee*: During mid-stance the knee reaches its peak of stance phase flexion and starts to extend again (Fig. 2.5), initially through concentric contraction of the quadriceps. The peak generally occurs at between 15 and 20 per cent of the gait cycle. Its magnitude is variable, both from one individual to another and with the speed of walking, but it is commonly between 10° and 20°.

5. *Ankle and foot*: The mid-stance rocker, also called the second rocker or ankle rocker, occurs during mid-stance and terminal stance. It is characterized by forward rotation of the tibia about the ankle joint as the foot remains flat on the floor, the ankle angle changing from plantar-flexion to dorsiflexion, with the triceps surae contracting eccentrically. The actual angles vary with the method of measurement; most authors report larger angles than those seen in Fig. 2.5. External rotation of the tibia and coupled forefoot supination occur during mid-stance and terminal stance. The ground reaction force vector moves forward along the foot from the time of foot flat onwards, moving into the forefoot prior to heel rise. The movement of the forefoot into supination peaks in mid-stance, and then begins to reverse towards pronation.

6. *Moments and powers*: During mid-stance the internal extensor moment at the hip, generated by contraction of the extensor muscles, declines and disappears, to be replaced by a moment in the opposite direction (Fig. 2.6). At the knee the force vector remains behind the joint,

Figure 2.14 Heel rise position of right leg (solid line), left leg (dashed line) and ground reaction force vector.

producing an external flexor moment, opposed by an internal extensor moment (Fig. 2.6), due to quadriceps contraction (Fig. 2.9). According to Perry (1992), only the vasti and not the rectus femoris are active at this time. As the direction of knee motion changes from flexion to extension (Fig. 2.5), power generation takes place (K2 in Fig. 2.6). The ankle shows an increasing internal plantarflexor moment throughout mid-stance and into terminal stance (Fig. 2.6) as the force vector moves into the forefoot. This moment is generated by the triceps surae (Fig. 2.9) contracting eccentrically and absorbing power (A1 in Fig. 2.7).

Heel rise (Fig. 2.14)

1. *General*: Heel rise, also called heel off, marks the transition from mid-stance to terminal stance. It is the time at which the heel begins to lift from the walking surface. Its timing varies considerably, both from one individual to another and with the speed of walking. The subject used for illustration showed heel rise at 32 per cent of the gait cycle.
2. *Upper body*: By heel rise, the trunk is falling from its highest point, reached during mid-stance. The lateral displacement over the supporting (right) leg also begins to diminish in preparation for the transfer of weight back to the left leg. As the right hip extends and the leg moves backwards, the right side of the pelvis twists backwards with it, and the arms and shoulder girdle on the right move forwards.
3. *Hip*: At heel rise and into terminal stance, the hip continues to extend (Fig. 2.5). Peak hip extension is reached around the time of opposite initial contact. The activity of the hip abductors in the frontal plane is still required, to stabilize the pelvis, although this activity ceases prior to initial contact by the other foot.
4. *Knee*: The knee has an extension peak close to the time of heel rise (Fig. 2.5). Around this time, active ankle plantarflexion brings the ground reaction force forward, moving it into the forefoot and in front of the knee joint (barely visible in Fig. 2.14). This attempts to extend the knee, an effect known as the plantarflexion/knee extension couple. Contraction of the gastrocnemius augments the action of the soleus as far as the ankle joint is concerned, but it also acts as a flexor at the knee, preventing hyperextension and subsequently initiating knee flexion.
5. *Ankle and foot*: The peak of ankle dorsiflexion is reached some time after heel rise (Fig. 2.5). Triceps surae initially maintains the ankle angle as the knee begins to flex, with movement into plantarflexion only beginning late in terminal stance. The tibia becomes increasingly externally rotated and the forefoot becomes increasingly supinated, the two being linked through coupled motion at the subtalar joint. As the heel rises, the toes remain flat on the ground and extension occurs at the metatarsophalangeal (MTP) joints, along an oblique line across the foot known as the metatarsal break or toe break. From the time that the heel rises, hindfoot inversion (adduction or varus angulation) is seen.
6. *Moments and powers*: At heel rise there is a small but increasing internal hip flexor moment (Fig. 2.6). The source of this internal flexor moment does not appear to have been fully explained in the literature,

Figure 2.15 Opposite initial contact position of right leg (solid line), left leg (dashed line) and ground reaction force vector.

although it could be due to a combination of adductor longus and rectus femoris contraction, and stretching of ligaments as the hip moves into extension, with a resulting power absorption (H2 in Fig. 2.7). At the knee, quadriceps contraction has ceased prior to heel rise, and the internal knee moment has reversed to become flexor. According to Perry (1992), this occurs because the upper body moves forward faster than the tibia. If the ankle joint were totally free, the forward motion of the body would simply dorsiflex the ankle. However, contraction of the triceps surae (Fig. 2.9) slows down the forward motion of the tibia, so that as the femur moves forwards an external extensor moment is generated at the knee, opposed by an internal flexor moment (Fig. 2.6). Only small and variable power exchanges occur at the knee around heel rise. At the ankle the internal dorsiflexor moment continues to increase, as first the soleus and then both soleus and gastrocnemius together (triceps surae in Fig. 2.9) contract increasingly strongly. The contraction is initially eccentric, with power absorption (A1 in Fig. 2.7).

Opposite initial contact (Fig. 2.15)

1. *General*: As might be expected, opposite initial contact in symmetrical gait occurs at close to 50 per cent of the cycle. It marks the end of the period of single support and the beginning of pre-swing, which is the second period of double support. At the time of opposite initial contact, also known as opposite foot contact, the hip begins to flex, the knee is flexing, and the ankle is plantarflexing. The period between heel rise and toe off, consisting of terminal stance followed by pre-swing, is sometimes called the terminal rocker. This is appropriate, since the leg is now rotating forwards about the forefoot rather than about the ankle joint. Another term for this period is the 'push-off' phase. Perry (1974)

objected to this term, suggesting instead the term 'roll-off', because 'the late floor-reaction peak is the result of leverage by body alignment, rather than an active downward thrust'. However, it is clear that the 'push off' is not simply passive, since it is the period during which the generation of power at the ankle is greatest (Winter, 1983). What is not clear is whether this power is used to accelerate the whole body (as suggested by Winter) or merely the leg (as suggested by Perry), or (as seems most likely) some combination of the two.

2. *Upper body*: The attitude of the upper body at opposite initial contact resembles that described for initial contact, except that the trunk is now moving towards the left rather than the right, and the trunk is twisted so that the right shoulder and arm and the left side of the pelvis are forward.

3. *Hip*: At opposite initial contact the hip reaches its most extended position (typically between 10° and 20° of extension, depending on how it is measured), and motion reverses in the direction of flexion (Fig. 2.5). With the hip extended, adductor longus acts as the primary hip flexor (Perry, 1992) and probably generates sufficient moment to initiate hip flexion, particularly when combined with tension in the stretched hip ligaments and the effects of gravity.

4. *Knee*: The knee is already moving into flexion by the time of opposite initial contact (Fig. 2.5). The force vector has moved behind the knee, aiding its flexion (Fig. 2.15), and rectus femoris begins to contract eccentrically (included with quadriceps in Fig. 2.9) to prevent flexion from occurring too rapidly.

5. *Ankle and foot*: From before opposite initial contact until the foot leaves the ground at toe off, the ankle is moving into plantarflexion (Fig. 2.5) due to concentric contraction of the triceps surae (Fig. 2.9). Extension of the toes at the MTP joints continues, and causes a tightening of the plantar fascia. The forefoot reaches its maximal supination, with coupled external tibial rotation. Hindfoot inversion (adduction or varus angulation) is also present. These various factors combine to lock the midtarsal joints, resulting in high stability of the foot for loadbearing (Inman *et al.*, 1981; Rose and Gamble, 1994).

6. *Moments and powers*: A peak of hip internal flexor moment occurs around opposite initial contact (Fig. 2.6). As stated above (Opposite initial contact, section 3), it probably results from a combination of adductor longus contraction, passive tension in the hip ligaments, and gravity. As the direction of hip motion reverses from extension to flexion, power absorption (H2 in Fig. 2.7) is replaced by power generation (H3 in Fig. 2.7). During terminal stance, flexion of the knee brings the joint in front of the force vector (Fig. 2.15), reversing the external moment from extensor to flexor and hence changing the internal moment from flexor to extensor (Fig. 2.6). Eccentric contraction of rectus femoris (included with quadriceps in Fig. 2.9) limits the rate of knee flexion, and results in power absorption (K3 in Fig. 2.7). At the ankle, the force vector is well in front of the joint at opposite initial contact (Fig. 2.15). The resulting high external dorsiflexor moment is opposed by a corresponding internal plantarflexor moment (Fig. 2.6), produced by concentric contraction of the triceps surae (Fig. 2.9). The result is a large

Figure 2.16 Toe off position of right leg (solid line), left leg (dashed line) and ground reaction force vector.

generation of power (A2 in Fig. 2.7), which represents the highest generation of power during the entire gait cycle.

Toe off (Fig. 2.16)

1. *General*: Toe off generally occurs at about 60 per cent of the gait cycle (57 per cent in the subject used for illustration). It separates pre-swing from initial swing, and is the point at which the stance phase ends and the swing phase begins. The name 'terminal contact' has been proposed for this event, since in pathological gait the toe may not be the last part of the foot to leave the ground.
2. *Upper body*: The extreme rotations of the shoulders, arms and trunk all begin to return towards the neutral position as the trunk gains height and moves towards the new (left) supporting foot.
3. *Hip*: As the foot leaves the ground, the hip continues to flex (Fig. 2.5). This is achieved by gravity and tension in the hip ligaments, as well as by contraction of the rectus femoris (included with quadriceps in Fig. 2.9) and adductor longus.
4. *Knee*: By the time of toe off, the knee has flexed to around half of the angle it will achieve at the peak of swing phase flexion. This flexion is aided by the positioning of the ground reaction force vector well behind the knee (Fig. 2.16), although the magnitude of the force declines rapidly, reaching zero as the foot leaves the ground. The major part of knee flexion then results from hip flexion: the leg acts as a jointed double pendulum, so that as the hip flexes the shank is 'left behind' due to its inertia, resulting in flexion of the knee. At the very beginning of the swing phase rectus femoris contracts eccentrically to prevent excessive knee flexion, particularly at faster walking speeds (Nene *et al.*, 1999).
5. *Ankle and foot*: The peak of ankle plantarflexion occurs just after toe

Figure 2.17 Feet adjacent position of right leg (solid line) and left leg (dashed line).

off. The magnitude of plantarflexion depends on how it is measured; it is 25° in Fig. 2.5. Triceps surae contraction ceases prior to toe off, and tibialis anterior begins to contract (Fig. 2.9) to bring the ankle up into a neutral or dorsiflexed attitude during the swing phase.

6. *Moments and powers*: Around toe off the hip still shows an internal flexor moment (Fig. 2.6), resulting from gravity, ligament elasticity, and adductor longus and iliopsoas contraction. Since the hip is flexing at this time, power generation occurs (H3 in Fig. 2.7). As stated above (Toe off, section 4), during pre-swing and initial swing, hip flexion causes the knee to flex, the double pendulum resulting in an external flexor moment at the knee opposed by an internal extensor moment (Fig. 2.6) as rectus femoris contracts eccentrically (included with quadriceps in Fig. 2.9) to limit the speed at which the knee flexes. This eccentric contraction absorbs power (K3 in Fig. 2.7). At the ankle, the internal plantarflexor moment reduces rapidly during terminal support as the magnitude of the ground reaction force declines, falling to zero as the foot leaves the ground at toe off (Fig. 2.6). The ankle power generation peak also declines to around zero during this period (Fig. 2.7).

Feet adjacent (Fig. 2.17)

1. *General*: Feet adjacent separates initial swing from mid-swing. It is the time when the swinging leg passes the stance phase leg, and the two feet are side by side. The swing phase occupies about 40 per cent of the gait cycle, and the feet become adjacent around the center of this time; in the subject used for illustration it occurred at 77 per cent of the gait cycle. Alternative names for feet adjacent are foot clearance and mid-swing; the latter term is now applied to a period of the gait cycle rather than to an event. Initial swing is also known as lift off.

2. *Upper body*: When the feet are adjacent, the trunk is at its highest position and is maximally displaced over the stance phase leg (left). The arms are level with each other, one (left) moving forward and one (right) moving back.

3. *Hip*: The hip starts to flex even prior to toe off, and by the time the feet are adjacent it is well flexed (20° in Fig. 2.5). This is achieved by a powerful contraction of iliopsoas (Fig. 2.9), aided by gravity.

4. *Knee*: The flexion of the knee during the swing phase results largely from the flexion of the hip. As described above (Toe off, section 6), the leg acts as a jointed pendulum, and no muscular contraction is necessary around the knee (thus enabling above-knee amputees to achieve swing phase knee flexion in their prosthetic limb). The peak swing phase knee flexion angle is usually between 60° and 70°. It occurs before the feet are adjacent, by which time the knee has started to extend again.

5. *Ankle and foot*: At the time the feet are adjacent, the ankle is moving from a plantarflexed attitude around toe off towards a neutral or dorsiflexed attitude in terminal swing. Most of the shortening of the swing phase leg required to achieve toe clearance comes from flexion of the knee, but the ankle also needs to move out of plantarflexion. This movement requires contraction of the anterior tibial muscles, although the force of contraction is much less than that required to control foot lowering following initial contact. The closest approach of the toes to the ground occurs around the time the feet are adjacent. In normal walking the toes clear the ground by very little; Murray (1967) found a mean clearance of 14 mm with a range of 1–38 mm. The degree of forefoot supination reduces following toe off, but the forefoot remains slightly supinated until the following initial contact.

6. *Moments and powers*: As the hip moves into flexion, from opposite

Figure 2.18 Tibia vertical position of right leg (solid line) and left leg (dashed line).

initial contact, through pre-swing and initial swing until the feet are adjacent, an internal flexor moment is present (Fig. 2.6). This is generated by gravity, rectus femoris and the adductors, with the addition of ligament elasticity at the beginning of the movement and iliopsoas contraction towards its end (Fig. 2.9). Hip flexion, in response to this moment, results in the highest peak of power generation at the hip (H3 in Fig. 2.7), the power being used to accelerate the swinging leg forward. The resulting kinetic energy is later transferred to the trunk, as the swinging leg is decelerated again at the end of the swing phase. Between toe off and feet adjacent, the knee continues to show a small internal extensor moment, as rectus femoris (part of quadriceps in Fig. 2.9) prevents the knee from flexing too rapidly in response to the external flexor moment transferred from the hip (see above). While the knee is still flexing, power absorption occurs (K3 in Fig. 2.7). Only very small moments and power exchanges are seen at the ankle, since only the weight of the foot is involved.

Tibia vertical (Fig. 2.18)·

1. *General*: The division between the periods of mid-swing and terminal swing is marked by the tibia of the swinging leg becoming vertical, which occurred at 86 per cent of the gait cycle in the subject used for illustration. Terminal swing is also known as reach.
2. *Upper body*: When the tibia is vertical on the swing phase leg (right), the trunk has begun to lose vertical height and to move from its maximum displacement over the supporting (left) leg back towards the midline. The left arm is now in front of the right, and the right side of the pelvis is a little in front of the left side (Fig. 2.18).
3. *Hip*: Tibia vertical marks approximately the time at which further hip flexion ceases, the subject used for illustration having a hip angle of about 27° of flexion from tibia vertical to the next initial contact (Fig. 2.5). The hamstrings contract increasingly strongly during terminal swing (Fig. 2.9), to limit the rate of knee extension, while maintaining the hip joint in this flexed position.
4. *Knee*: Tibia vertical occurs during a period of rapid knee extension, as the knee goes from the peak of swing phase flexion, prior to feet adjacent, to more-or-less full extension prior to the next initial contact (Fig. 2.5). This extension is largely passive, being the return swing of the lower (shank) segment of the double pendulum referred to above (Toe off, section 6). Eccentric contraction of the hamstrings prevents this motion from causing an abrupt hyperextension of the knee at the end of swing (Fig. 2.9).
5. *Ankle and foot*: Once toe clearance has occurred, generally before the tibia becomes vertical, the ankle attitude becomes less important: it may be anywhere between a few degrees plantarflexed and a few degrees dorsiflexed, prior to the next initial contact (Fig. 2.5). Tibialis anterior continues to contract to hold the ankle in position, but its activity usually increases prior to initial contact in anticipation of the greater contraction forces that will be needed during the loading response (Fig. 2.9).

Figure 2.19 Lateral, fore–aft and vertical components of the ground reaction force, in newtons, for right foot (solid line) and left foot (dashed line). Abbreviations as in Fig. 2.5. See text for sign conventions.

6. *Moments and powers:* At the hip, by the time of tibia vertical an increasing internal extensor moment is seen (Fig. 2.6), largely generated by contraction of the hamstrings, although gluteus maximus also begins to contract prior to the next initial contact (Fig. 2.9). This moment probably permits the transfer of momentum from the swinging leg to the trunk, recovering some of the kinetic energy imparted to the leg in initial swing (H3 in Fig. 2.7). Since the hip angle is essentially static during terminal swing, very little power exchange occurs at the joint itself. The knee demonstrates an increasing internal flexor moment (Fig. 2.6), which is generated by eccentric contraction of the hamstrings (Fig. 2.9), with power absorption (K4 in Fig. 2.7). This occurs in response to an external extensor moment, generated by the inertia of the swinging shank, which would hyperextend the knee if it was not checked. The ankle moment remains negligible (Fig. 2.6), with very little power exchange (Fig. 2.7).

Terminal foot contact (Fig. 2.10)

The gait cycle ends at the next initial contact of the same foot (in this case, the right foot). Because it is confusing to refer to the *end* of the cycle as 'initial contact', it is sometimes known as terminal foot contact.

Ground reaction forces

The *force platform* (or forceplate) is an instrument commonly used in gait analysis. It gives the total force applied by the foot to the ground, although it does not show the distribution of different parts of this force (e.g. heel and forefoot) on the walking surface. Some force platforms give only one component of the force (usually vertical), but most give a full three-dimensional description of the ground reaction force vector. The electrical output signals may be processed to produce three components of force (vertical, lateral and fore-aft), the two coordinates of the center of pressure, and the moments about the vertical axis. The *center of pressure* is the point on the ground through which a single resultant force appears to act, although in reality the total force is made up of innumerable small force vectors spread over a finite area on the surface of the platform.

Since the ground reaction force is a three-dimensional vector, it would be preferable to display it as such for the purposes of interpretation. Unfortunately, this is seldom practical. The most common form of display is that shown in Fig. 2.19, where the three components of force are plotted against time, for the walk shown in the previous Figs. The sign convention used in Fig. 2.19 is the same as that used by Winter (1991), where the ground reaction force is positive upwards, forwards and to the right. Regrettably, there is no general agreement on sign conventions.

The lateral component of force is generally very small; for most of the stance phase of the right foot the ground reaction force accelerates the center of gravity towards the left side of the body, and during the stance phase of the left foot the acceleration is towards the right side of the body. The fore–aft (or antero-posterior) trace from the right foot shows 'braking' during the first half of the stance phase and 'propulsion' during the second half. The left foot shows the same pattern, but with the direction of the lateral force reversed. The vertical force shows a characteristic double hump, which results from an upward acceleration of the center of gravity during early stance, a reduction in downward force as the body 'flies' over the leg in mid-stance, and a second peak due to deceleration, as the downward motion is checked in late stance.

Plots of this type are difficult to interpret, and encourage consideration of the force vector as separate components rather than as a three-dimensional whole. The butterfly diagram shown in Fig. 2.8 is an improvement on this, since it combines two of the force components (vertical and fore–aft) with the fore–aft coordinate of the center of pressure. It also preserves information on timing, since the lines representing the force vector are at regular intervals (10 ms in this case). Butterfly diagrams for the frontal and transverse planes are more difficult to interpret, and are seldom used.

The other type of information commonly derived from the force platform is the position of the center of pressure of the two feet on the ground, as shown in Fig. 2.20, again for the same walk. This may be used to identify abnormal patterns of foot contact, including an abnormal toe out or toe in angle. The step length and walking base can also be measured from this type of display, providing there is an identifiable initial contact.

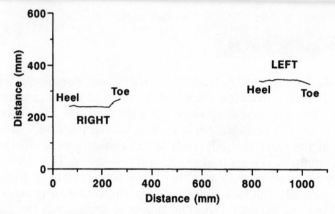

Figure 2.20 View of the walking surface from above, showing the center of pressure beneath the two feet, with the right heel contacting first and the subject walking towards the right of the diagram.

If the pattern of foot contact is of particular interest, it is preferable to combine the data on the center of pressure with an outline of the foot obtained by some other means (such as chalk on the floor). This type of display, with the addition of a sagittal plane representation of the ground reaction force vector, is shown in Fig. 2.21 for a normal male subject wearing shoes. The trace shows initial contact at the back of the heel on the lateral side, with progression of the center of force along the middle of the foot to the metatarsal heads, where it moves medially, ending at the hallux. The spacing of the vectors shows how long the center of pressure spends in any one area. It is worth noting that there is a cluster of vectors just in front of the edge of the heel, where the shoe is not in contact with the ground, again pointing out the fact that the center of pressure is merely the average of a number of forces acting beneath the foot.

There is considerable variation between individuals as to how much force is applied to the ground at initial contact, some people 'gliding' the foot onto the ground and others 'digging' it in. Fig. 2.22 shows the vertical component of the ground reaction force from a fast walk, in hard-heeled shoes, by an individual with a marked heelstrike. The data were recorded at 1000 Hz from a Bertec force platform, which has a particularly high frequency response. It has been suggested that transient forces in the joints, resulting from the heelstrike, may cause degenerative arthritis (Radin, 1987). The heelstrike transient represents the transfer of momentum from the moving leg to the ground. It is a fairly short event, typically lasting 10–20 ms, and can only be observed using measuring equipment with a fast enough response time.

Moments about the vertical axis are seldom reported. In comparing these moments between normal children with children with clubfeet, Sawatzky *et al.* (1994) were surprised to find only small, and not statistically significant, differences. However, as will be explained in Chapter 4, these moments largely result from the acceleration and deceleration of the swing phase leg, and only minor changes could be expected to be introduced by the foot.

Figure 2.21 Foot outline, center of pressure and sagittal plane representation of ground reaction force vector; right foot of a normal male subject walking in shoes.

Figure 2.22 Plot of vertical ground reaction force against time, showing the heelstrike transient in a particularly vigorous walker wearing hard-heeled shoes. Unfiltered data from Bertec force platform, sampled at 1000 Hz.

Support moment

Winter (1980) coined the term 'support moment' to describe the sum of the sagittal plane moments about the hip, knee and ankle joints:

$$M_S = M_H + M_K + M_A$$

where M_S, M_H, M_K and M_A are the support, hip, knee and ankle moments, respectively.

Winter noted that the support moment was far less variable than its individual components, suggesting that a decreased moment about one

Figure 2.23 Support moment, calculated using the formula of Hof (2000), from the sagittal plane internal joint moments of right hip, knee and ankle. Abbreviations and sign conventions as in Figs 2.5 and 2.6.

joint could be compensated for by an increased moment about one or both of the other joints. However, it was difficult to interpret this in biomechanical terms because the sign convention was based on flexion and extension rather than on clockwise and counterclockwise moments, so that the direction of the knee moment was opposite to that of the hip and ankle moments. Hof (2000) published a justification for the support moment, and suggested that it is responsible for preventing collapse of the knee. Based on his analysis, he suggested the following revised formula for its calculation:

$$M_S = \tfrac{1}{2}M_H + M_K + \tfrac{1}{2}M_A$$

Fig. 2.23 illustrates the support moment, calculated from the sagittal plane hip, knee and ankle internal moments from the normal subject used for illustration throughout this chapter, using the formula suggested by Hof (2000).

Energy consumption

It is relatively easy to measure the energy consumption of a vehicle, but much more difficult to make equivalent measurements of human walking, for two reasons. First, there is a clear relationship between the fuel level in the tank of a vehicle and how much energy has been used, whereas knowing how much food a person has eaten gives no information on the energy consumed in a particular activity. Secondly, a vehicle that is switched off uses no energy, whereas people use metabolic energy all the time, whether they are walking or not.

The first problem, that of measuring the 'fuel consumption', can be solved by measuring not the fuel consumed but the oxygen that is used to oxidize it. Measurements of oxygen uptake, while not particularly pleasant for the subject (who has to wear a face mask or mouthpiece), are nonetheless perfectly practical, and are used routinely to measure the metabolic cost of different activities.

The second problem, the lack of a suitable baseline for energy consumption measurements in humans, is not easy to solve and requires a different way of thinking about the topic. The energy used by a person who is walking can be divided into three parts:

1. The muscles used for walking consume energy as they accelerate and decelerate the trunk and the limb segments in different directions.
2. There is an 'overhead' involved in walking, in that the expenditure of energy by the muscles involves increased activity by the heart and the muscles used in breathing, which themselves use energy. Energy is also expended in maintaining the upright posture.
3. The basal metabolism is the irreducible minimum energy a person will consume if they are totally at rest.

The relationship between metabolic energy and physical energy is very complicated. As explained in Chapter 1, if a muscle undergoes an isometric contraction it still uses energy, although its length does not change and the physical work it does is zero. In an eccentric contraction, when it lengthens under tension, it uses up metabolic energy when in physical terms it would be expected to gain energy rather than to lose it.

In the past it has been usual to estimate the mechanical efficiency of walking by looking at the difference in oxygen consumption between the basal state and walking at a given speed. This approach neglects the various overheads, however, and makes slow walking appear to be extremely inefficient. Inman *et al.* (1981) and Rose and Gamble (1994) suggested that it is more realistic to use standing or very slow walking as the baseline for measurements on faster walking. Despite these uncertainties, a figure of 25 per cent is often quoted for the efficiency of the conversion of metabolic energy into mechanical energy in a wide range of activities, including walking. A comprehensive review of the energy expenditure of normal and pathological gait was given by Waters and Mulroy (1999).

The energy requirements of walking can be expressed in two ways: the energy used per unit time, and the energy used per unit distance. Since energy expenditure is usually inferred from the oxygen used, these are generally known as oxygen consumption and oxygen cost, respectively.

Energy consumption per unit time

Inman *et al.* (1981) and Rose and Gamble (1994) quoted an equation, based on a number of studies, for the relationship between the walking speed and the energy consumption per unit time. The energy consumption included both the basal metabolism and the 'overheads'. They showed, not surprisingly, that energy consumption per unit time is less for slow walking than for fast walking. Translating their equation into SI units, it becomes:

$$E_w = 2.23 + 1.26v^2$$

where E_w is the energy consumption in watts per kilogram body mass, and v is the speed in m/s.

As an example of the application of this equation, a 70 kg person walking at 1.4 m/s, which is a typical speed for adults, would consume energy at a rate of 330 W.

Energy consumption per unit distance

The energy consumption per meter walked, also known as 'energy cost', and related to 'oxygen cost', has a less straightforward relationship with walking speed, as both very slow and very fast walking speeds use more energy per meter than walking at intermediate speeds. The equation that describes this relationship, again converted into SI units, is:

$$E_m = 2.23/v + 1.26v$$

where E_m is the energy consumption in joules per meter per kilogram body mass, and v is the speed in m/s.

The minimum energy usage is predicted by this equation at a speed of 1.33 m/s. A 70 kg person walking at this speed would use 235 joules per meter, or 235 kJ per kilometer. A typical candy bar contains around 1000 kJ, and would thus supply enough energy to walk 4.26 km, or more than two and a half miles!

The equations quoted above merely give average values for adults, which may be modified by age, sex, walking surface, footwear and so on. Pathological gait is frequently associated with an energy consumption considerably above these 'average' values, due to some combination of abnormal movements, muscle spasticity and co-contraction of antagonistic muscles. To provide a baseline for studies of pathological gait, Waters *et al.* (1988) made a detailed study of the energy consumption of a total of 260 normal children and adults of both sexes, walking at a variety of speeds.

Optimization of energy usage

If people were fitted with wheels, very little energy would be needed for locomotion on a level surface, and some of the energy expended in going uphill would be recovered when coming down again. For this reason, both wheelchairs and bicycles are remarkably efficient forms of transport, although obviously much less versatile than a pair of legs. During walking, each leg in turn has to be started and stopped, and the center of gravity of the body rises and falls and moves from side to side, all of which use energy. Despite this, walking is not as inefficient as it might be due to two forms of optimization – those involving transfers of energy, and those that minimize the displacement of the center of gravity.

Energy transfers

Two types of energy transfer occur during walking – an exchange between potential and kinetic energy, and the transfer of energy between one limb segment and another. The most obvious exchange between potential and kinetic energy is in the movement of the trunk. During the double support phase, the trunk is at its lowest vertical position with its highest forward speed. During the first half of the single support phase the trunk is lifted up by the supporting leg, converting some of its kinetic energy into potential energy as its speed reduces. During the latter part of the single support phase the trunk drops down again, in front of the supporting leg, and reduces its height while picking up speed again. These exchanges between potential and kinetic energy are the same as in a child's swing, in which the potential energy at the highest point in its travel is converted into kinetic energy as it swings downwards, then back into potential energy again as it swings up the other side.

As well as the vertical motion of the trunk, there are other exchanges between potential and kinetic energy in walking. The twisting of the shoulder girdle and pelvis in opposite directions stores potential energy as tension in the elastic structures, which is converted to kinetic energy as the trunk untwists, and then back to potential energy again as the trunk twists the other way.

Winter *et al.* (1976) studied the energy levels of the limb segments and of the quaintly named HAT (Head, Arms and Trunk). These authors criticized some earlier studies, which had included the kinetic energy of linear motion but neglected the kinetic energy due to rotation, which is respons-ible for about 10 per cent of the total energy of the shank. Winter *et al.* studied only the sagittal plane, regarding energy exchanges in the other planes as negligible. They confirmed the exchange between potential and kinetic energy, described above, and estimated that roughly half of the energy of the HAT segment was conserved in this way. The thigh conserved about a third of its energy by exchanges of this sort, and the shank virtually none. They also noted that the changes in total body energy were less than the changes in energy of the individual segments, indicating a transfer of energy from one segment to another. In one subject, during a single gait cycle, the energy changes were: shank 16 J, thigh 6 J and HAT 10 J, making a total of 32 J. However, the total body energy change was only 22 J, indicating a saving of 10 J by inter-segment transfers.

The six determinants of gait

The six optimizations used to minimize the excursions of the center of gravity were called the determinants of gait by Saunders *et al.* (1953) in a classic paper, the main points of which were reiterated, with slight

Figure 2.24 First determinant of gait: if the pelvis did not rotate (left), the whole of the stride length would come from hip flexion and extension. Pelvic rotation about a vertical axis (right) reduces the angle of hip flexion and extension, which in turn reduces the vertical movement of the hip.

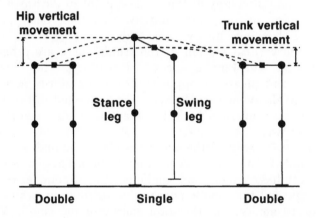

Figure 2.25 Second determinant of gait: the vertical movement of the trunk is less than that of the hip, due to pelvic tilt about an anteroposterior axis.

changes, by Inman *et al.* (1981) and Rose and Gamble (1994). A brief description is given below, but one of these sources should be consulted for a detailed and well-illustrated account. The fourth and fifth determinants were combined in the original descriptions, but for the purposes of clarity the present author has separated them and made other minor changes.

For more than 40 years since their first publication, the determinants of gait were generally accepted, and have been re-described in numerous publications – including the first two editions of the present book. However, it has recently been suggested in a series of publications (e.g. Gard and Childress, 1997) that the second and third determinants of gait (pelvic obliquity and knee flexion in stance) play little or no part in reducing energy expenditure. Although these motions certainly occur, the reason for their existence may not be as originally described. However,

Initial contact   Stance phase knee flexion   Heel rise   Toe off

Figure 2.26 Third, fourth and fifth determinants of gait: stance phase knee flexion shortens the leg in mid-stance (third determinant); backward projection of the heel at initial contact lengthens the leg (fourth determinant); so does forward projection of the forefoot during pre-swing (fifth determinant).

having provided this warning, I will nonetheless reiterate the original descriptions!

The six 'determinants of gait' are as follows:

1. *Pelvic rotation*: If the knee is kept straight, a movement of the hip from a flexed position to an extended one (such as occurs in the stance phase of gait) will result in the hip joint moving forwards, but also in its rising and then falling again. The amount of forward movement and the amount of rising and falling both depend on the total angle the hip joint moves through from flexion to extension (Fig. 2.24, left). Since the forward movement is equal to the stride length, it follows that the greater the stride length, the greater will be the angles of flexion and extension of the hip, and the more the hip will move vertically between its highest and lowest positions. The first determinant of gait is the way in which the pelvis twists about a vertical axis during the gait cycle, bringing each hip joint forwards as that hip flexes and backwards as it extends. This means that for a given stride length, less flexion and extension of the hip is required, since a proportion of the stride length comes from the forward and backward movement of the hip joint rather than the angular movement of the leg. The reduction in the range of hip flexion and extension leads to a reduction in the vertical movement of the hip (Fig. 2.24, right).
2. *Pelvic obliquity*: As described above, flexion and extension of the hip are accompanied by a rise and fall in the height of the hip joint. If the pelvis were to keep level, the trunk would follow this up-and-down movement. However, the second determinant of gait is the way in which the pelvis tips about an antero-posterior axis, raising first one side and then the other, so that when the hip of the stance phase leg is at its highest point the pelvis slopes downwards so that the hip of the swing phase leg is lower than that of the stance phase leg. Since the height of the trunk does not depend on the height of either hip joint

Figure 2.27 Sixth determinant of gait: if the feet are placed on the ground far apart (a), large side-to-side movements of the center of gravity would be necessary to maintain balance; having them closer together (b) reduces the size of these movements.

alone, but on the average of the two of them, this pelvic obliquity reduces the total vertical excursion of the trunk (Fig. 2.25). However, it can only be achieved if the swing phase leg can be shortened sufficiently to clear the ground (normally by both flexing the knee and dorsiflexing the ankle), when the height of its hip joint is reduced.

3. *Knee flexion in stance phase*: The third, fourth and fifth determinants of gait (Fig. 2.26) are all concerned with adjusting the effective length of the leg, by lengthening it at the beginning and end of the stance phase and shortening it in the middle, to keep the hip height as constant as possible. The third determinant is the stance phase flexion of the knee. As the femur passes from flexion of the hip into extension, if the leg remained straight the hip joint would rise and then fall. However, flexion of the knee shortens the leg in the middle of this movement, reducing the height of the apex of the curve.

4. *Ankle mechanism*: Complementary to the way in which the apex of the curve is lowered by shortening the leg in the middle of the movement from hip flexion to extension, the beginning of the curve is elevated by lengthening the leg at the start of the stance phase – initial contact. This is achieved by the fourth determinant of gait – the ankle mechanism. Because the heel sticks out behind the ankle joint, it effectively lengthens the leg during the loading response (Fig. 2.26).

5. *Foot mechanism*: In the same way that the heel lengthens the leg at the start of the stance phase, the forefoot lengthens it at the end of stance, in the fifth determinant – the terminal rocker (Fig. 2.26). From the time of

heel rise, the effective length of the lower leg increases as the ankle moves from dorsiflexion into plantarflexion.

6. *Lateral displacement of body*: The first five determinants of gait are all concerned with reducing the vertical excursions of the center of gravity. The sixth is concerned with side-to-side movement. If the feet were as far apart as the hips, the body would need to tip from side to side to maintain balance during walking (Fig. 2.27a). By keeping the walking base narrow, little lateral movement is needed to preserve balance (Fig. 2.27b). The reduction in lateral acceleration and deceleration leads to a reduction in the use of muscular energy. The main adaptation that allows the walking base to be narrow is a slight valgus angulation of the knee, which permits the tibia to be vertical while the femur inclines inwards from a slightly adducted hip.

It should be obvious that although the six determinants of gait have been described separately, they are all integrated together during each gait cycle. The combined effect is a much smoother trajectory for the center of gravity and a much reduced energy expenditure than would have been the case without them. According to Perry (1992), the determinants of gait reduce the vertical excursions of the trunk by about 50 per cent and the horizontal excursions by about 40 per cent.

Starting and stopping

To this point, only steady state continuous walking has been considered. In order to achieve that state the individual has to start off and, on reaching the destination, to stop. Winter (1995), in a review of balance and posture control, gave a good description of gait initiation and gait termination.

In gait initiation, from standing on both feet the body weight is shifted to one foot, thus permitting the other foot to be lifted off the ground and moved forward. As an example, suppose the left foot was going to move forwards first (swing limb) while the body weight is supported by the right foot (stance limb). The shifting of weight over the right foot is achieved by a brief initial push, backwards and to the left, by the left foot. This (following Newton's second law) moves the center of gravity of the body forwards and to the right. Once the center of gravity is over the right foot, it is safe to lift the left foot off the ground and to move it forward. At the same time, the trunk has started to move forward. The left foot lands on the ground in front of the subject, with a step that is almost exactly the same as in steady state gait. Body weight is transferred to the left leg, the right foot leaves the ground with a normal toe off, and the subject is walking. By the time the left foot has contacted the ground the trunk is moving forward at around 85 per cent of the final walking speed, and only one or two more steps are needed before the steady state speed and pattern are achieved. Probably the slowest adjustment is that of side-to-side balance, which may need several steps to stabilize.

A pathology that causes particular problems for the initiation of gait is parkinsonism; gait initiation in this condition was reviewed by Halliday *et al.* (1998).

Less research has been done on gait termination, although it appears to present a greater challenge to the neural control system. Gait termination involves a stance phase on one side, which is not followed by a swing phase. On the other side, there is a shortened swing phase, the moving foot being placed beside the stationary one. If the left foot is the swinging one the forces to terminate gait are provided by the right foot, which directs the ground reaction force forward and to the right, thus applying a backwards and leftwards force to the body center of gravity, arresting its forward motion and bringing it to the mid-point between the feet. The left foot is then planted on the ground beside the right one, and the walk has terminated.

Other varieties of gait

As well as normal walking, humans walk backwards, skip, run, ascend and descend slopes and stairs, step over obstacles, and carry loads in their hands, on their backs or on their heads. Running has an extensive literature of its own, since it is such an important part of sports medicine. The other types of locomotion have all been studied to a greater or lesser extent, particularly because patients with abnormal neuromuscular systems frequently have greater problems with some of these other activities than they do with normal walking. However, such considerations are beyond the scope of this introductory text.

Gait in the young

Although a number of studies have been made of the development of gait in children, that by Sutherland *et al.* (1988) is one of the most detailed. The main ways in which the gait of small children differs from that of adults are as follows:

1. The walking base is wider
2. The stride length and speed are lower and the cycle time shorter (higher cadence)
3. Small children have no heelstrike, initial contact being made by the flat foot
4. There is very little stance phase knee flexion
5. The whole leg is externally rotated during the swing phase
6. There is an absence of reciprocal arm swinging.

These differences in gait mature at different rates. The characteristics numbered (3), (4) and (5) in the above list have changed to the adult pattern by the age of 2 years, and (1) and (6) by the age of 4 years. The cycle time, stride length and speed continue to change with growth, reaching normal adult values around the age of 15.

Most children commence walking within 3 months of their first birthday. Prior to this, even tiny babies will make reciprocal stepping motions if they

Figure 2.28 Sagittal plane hip, knee and ankle angles in 1-year-old children. The hip angle has been moved into extension by 15° to allow for a difference in measurement methods. Sign conventions and abbreviations as in Fig. 2.5 (based on data from Sutherland *et al.*, 1988).

are moved slowly forwards while held in the standing position with their feet on the ground. However, this is not true walking, as there is little attempt to take any weight on the legs.

Fig. 2.28, which is based on data from Sutherland *et al.* (1988), shows the average sagittal plane motion at the hip, knee and ankle joints in 49 children aged between 11 and 13 months. It should be compared with Fig. 2.5, which shows the same parameters for a normal adult female. Sutherland *et al.* only gave the timing of initial contact and toe off on the two sides, and used a different definition of hip angle – the data in Fig. 2.28 have been adjusted into extension by 15° to make them comparable with the other figures in this book.

The pattern of hip flexion and extension differs from that in adults in that the degree of extension is reduced, and the hip does not remain flexed for so long at the end of the swing phase.

The knee never fully extends, but this is seen at all ages in Sutherland's data, and may reflect the method of measurement. There is some stance phase knee flexion in infants, but it is both smaller in magnitude and occurs earlier than in adults. The flexion of the knee in the swing phase is also somewhat reduced at the age of 1 year (most adults have more swing phase flexion than is seen in Fig. 2.5).

Initial contact in small children is by the whole foot, heelstrike being replaced by foot flat. The ankle is plantarflexed at initial contact and remains so into the early stance phase, in contrast to the adult pattern, in which the ankle is approximately neutral at initial contact but moves rapidly into plantarflexion. The pattern of dorsiflexion followed by plantar-flexion through the remainder of the stance phase is essentially the same at all ages.

Since children are smaller than adults, it is not surprising that they walk with a shorter stride length and at a slower speed. Sutherland *et al.* (1988) showed that stride length is closely related to height, and that the ratio of stride length to stature is similar to that found in adults. The change in stride length with age mirrors the change in height, showing a rapid increase up to age 4 years and a slower increase thereafter. Todd *et al.* (1989) detailed the relationships between the height of children and their general gait parameters. Small children walk with a short cycle time (rapid cadence), the mean at the age of 1 year being about 0.70 s (171 steps/min). Cycle time increases with age, but is still around 0.85 s (141 steps/min) at 7 years, which is well below the typical adult values of 1.06 s (113 steps/min) for men and 1.02 s (118 steps/min) for women. The shorter cycle time partly compensates for the short stride length, and the speed ranged from 0.64 m/s at age 1 year to 1.14 m/s at 7 years, compared with the typical adult values of 1.46 m/s for males and 1.30 m/s for females. Sutherland did not report on the gait of children beyond the age of 7 years, and did not distinguish between the results from boys and girls. Appendix 1 gives the normal ranges for the general gait parameters in children, derived in part from Sutherland's data. However, values based on age alone may be mis-leading – stride length depends on both height and walking speed, both of which may be lower in children with a disability than in normal children of the same age.

As can be seen in Fig. 2.28, the swing phase occupies a smaller propor-tion of the gait cycle in very small children than in adults, which minimizes the time spent in the less stable condition of single-legged stance. The relative duration of the swing phase increases with age, reaching the adult proportion around the age of 4 years. There is symmetry between the two sides at all ages. Sutherland *et al.* (1988) related the width of the walking base to the width of the body at the top of the pelvis, using the somewhat confusing 'pelvic-span/ankle-spread' ratio. Changing the measurement units for the sake of clarity, the walking base is about 70 per cent of the pelvic width at the age of 1 year, falling to about 45 per cent by $3\frac{1}{2}$ years, at which level it remains until the age of 7 years. An average value for adults is not readily available, but it is probably less than 30 per cent.

At the very youngest ages, the EMG patterns showed that there is a tendency to activate most muscles for a higher proportion of the gait cycle than in adults. With the exception of the triceps surae, adult patterns are established for most muscles by the age of 2 years. Sutherland *et al.* (1988) found that children could be divided into two groups depending on whether the triceps surae was activated in a prolonged (infant) pattern or the normal (adult) pattern. Below 2 years of age, over 60 per cent of the children showed the infant pattern; the propor-tion dropped to below 30 per cent by 7 years. The authors speculated that this might relate to delayed myelination of the sensory branches of the peripheral nerves.

An excellent review of the main changes in gait that occur during childhood was given by Sutherland (1997). The gait of very small children (under the age of 2 years) was examined in detail by Grimshaw *et al.* (1998).

Gait in the elderly

A number of investigations have been made regarding the changes in gait that occur with advancing age, especially by Murray *et al.* (1969), who studied the gait of men up to the age of 87 years. The description that follows is confined to the effects of age on free-speed walking, although Murray *et al.* also examined fast walking. A companion paper (Murray *et al.*, 1970) studied the gait of women up to the age of 70. It did not provide as much information on the effects of age, but generally confirmed the observations made on males.

The gait of the elderly is subject to two influences – the effects of age itself, and the effects of pathological conditions, such as osteoarthritis and parkinsonism, which become more common with advancing age. Providing patients with pathological conditions are carefully excluded, the gait of the elderly appears to be simply a 'slowed down' version of the gait of younger adults. Murray *et al.* (1969) were careful to point out that 'the walking performance of older men did not resemble a pathological gait'.

Typically, the onset of age-related changes in gait takes place in the decade from 60 to 70 years of age. There is a decreased stride length, a variable but generally increased cycle time (decreased cadence), and an increase in the walking base. Many other changes can also be observed, such as a relative increase in the duration of the stance phase as a percentage of the gait cycle, but most of them are secondary to the changes in stride length, cycle time and walking base. The speed (stride length divided by cycle time) is almost always reduced in elderly people. Appendix 1 gives normal ranges for the general gait parameters up to the age of 80 years.

Some of the differences between the gait of the young and the elderly are apparent in Fig. 2.29, which is taken from Murray *et al.* (1969). These authors suggested that the purpose of the gait changes in the elderly is to improve the security of walking. Both decreasing the stride length and increasing the walking base make it easier to maintain balance while walking. Increasing the cycle time (reducing the cadence) leads to a reduction in the percentage of the gait cycle for which there is only single limb support, since the increase in cycle length is largely achieved by lengthening the stance phase and hence the double support time.

Changes in the angular excursions of the joints in the elderly include a reduction in the total range of hip flexion and extension, a reduction in swing phase knee flexion, and reduced ankle plantarflexion during the push off. However, all of these depend on both cycle time and stride length, and are probably within normal limits if these factors are taken into account. Nigg *et al.* (1994) confirmed these observations in a detailed

Figure 2.29 Body position at right initial contact in older men (left) and younger men (right) (Murray *et al.*, 1969).

study on three-dimensional joint ranges of motion in walking in male and female subjects from 20 to 79 years of age.

The vertical movement of the head is reduced and its lateral movement increased, probably secondary to the changes in stride length and walking base, respectively.

The trajectory of the toe over the ground is modified in old age, giving an improved ground clearance during the first half of the swing phase. This is probably another mechanism for improving security. The heel rises less during pre-swing and the foot attitude is closer to the horizontal at initial contact, both of these changes being related to the reduction in stride length. There is also an increase in the angle of toe out in elderly people, and changes in the posture and movements of the arms, the elbows being more flexed and the shoulders more extended. The reasons for these differences are not known.

The dividing line between normal and abnormal gait may be difficult to define in elderly people. A condition known as 'idiopathic gait disorder of the elderly' has been described, which is essentially an exaggeration of the gait changes that normally occur with age, and is characterized by a cautious attitude to walking, with a prolonged cycle time (low cadence), a short stride length and an increased step-to-step variability. A comprehensive review of the changes in gait with advancing age was given by Prince *et al.* (1997).

References and suggestions for further reading

Blanc Y, Balmer C, Landis T, Vingerhoets F. (1999) Temporal parameters and patterns of foot roll over during walking: normative data for healthy adults. *Gait and Posture* **10**: 97–108.

Bresler B, Frankel JP. (1950) The forces and moments in the leg during level walking. *American Society of Mechanical Engineers Transactions* **72**: 27–36.

Cavagna GA, Margaria R. (1966) Mechanics of walking. *Journal of Applied Physiology*, **21**: 271–278.

Gage JR. (1990) An overview of normal walking. *American Academy of Orthopedic Surgeons: Instructional Course Lectures* **39**: 291–303.

Gard SA, Childress DS. (1997) The effect of pelvic list on the vertical displacement of the trunk during normal walking. *Gait and Posture* **5**: 233–238.

Garrison FH. (1929) *An Introduction to the History of Medicine.* Philadelphia, PA: W.B. Saunders Co.

Grimshaw PN, Marques-Bruna P, Salo A, Messenger N. (1998) The 3-dimensional kinematics of the walking gait cycle of children aged between 10 and 24 months: cross-sectional and repeated measures. *Gait and Posture* **7**: 7–15.

Halliday SE, Winter DA, Frank JS *et al.* (1998) The initiation of gait in young, elderly and Parkinson's disease subjects. *Gait and Posture* **8**: 8–14.

Hof AL. (2000) On the interpretation of the support moment. *Gait and Posture* **12**: 196–199.

Inman VT, Ralston HJ, Todd F. (1981) *Human Walking.* Baltimore, MD: Williams Wilkins.

Macellari V, Giacomozzi C, Saggini R. (1999) Spatial–temporal parameters of gait: reference data and a statistical method for normality assessment. *Gait and Posture* **10**: 171–181.

Murray MP. (1967) Gait as a total pattern of movement. *American Journal of Physical Medicine* **46**: 290–333.

Murray MP, Kory RC, Clarkson BH. (1969) Walking patterns in healthy old men. *Journal of Gerontology* **24**: 169–178.

Murray MP, Kory RC, Sepic SB. (1970) Walking patterns of normal women. *Archives of Physical Medicine and Rehabilitation* **51**: 637–650.

Nene A, Mayagoitia R, Veltink P. (1999) Assessment of rectus femoris function during initial swing phase. *Gait and Posture,* **9**: 1–9.

Nigg BM, Fisher V, Ronsky JL. (1994) Gait characteristics as a function of age and gender. *Gait and Posture* **2**: 213–220.

Oeffinger D, Brauch B, Cranfill S *et al.* (1999) Comparison of gait with and without shoes in children. *Gait and Posture* **9**: 95–100.

Pathokinesiology Service and Physical Therapy Department (1993) *Observational Gait Analysis.* Downey, CA: Los Amigos Research and Education Institute.

Paul JP. (1965) *Bio-engineering Studies of the Forces transmitted by Joints. (II) Engineering Analysis. Biomechanics and Related Bioengineering Topics* (JP Kenedi, ed.), pp. 369–380. Oxford: Pergamon Press.

Paul JP. (1966) Forces transmitted by joints in the human body. *Proceedings of the Institute of Mechanical Engineers* **181**: 8–15.

Pedotti A. (1977) Simple equipment used in clinical practice for the evaluation of locomotion. *IEEE Transactions on Biomedical Engineering,* **BME-24**: 456–461.

Perry J. (1974) Kinesiology of lower extremity bracing. *Clinical Orthopaedics and Related Research* **102**: 18–31.

Perry J. (1992) *Gait Analysis: Normal and Pathological Function.* Thorofare, NJ: SLACK Incorporated.

Prince F, Winter DA, Stergiou P, Walt SE. (1994) Anticipatory control of upper body balance during human locomotion. *Gait and Posture* **2**: 19–25.

Prince F, Corriveau H, Hébert R, Winter DA. (1997) Gait in the elderly. *Gait and Posture* **5**: 128–135.

Radin EL. (1987) Osteoarthrosis: what is known about its prevention. *Clinical Orthopaedics and Related Research* **222**: 60–65.

Rose J, Gamble JG. (1994) *Human Walking*, 2nd edn. Baltimore, MA: Williams & Wilkins.

Saunders JBDM, Inman VT, Eberhart HS. (1953) The major determinants in normal and pathological gait. *Journal of Bone and Joint Surgery* **35A**: 543–558.

Sawatzky BJ, Sanderson DJ, Beauchamp RD, Outerbridge AR. (1994) Ground reaction forces in gait in children with clubfeet – a preliminary study. *Gait and Posture* **2**: 123–127.

Sekiya N, Nagasaki H. (1998) Reproducibility of the walking patterns of normal young adults: test–retest reliability of the walk ratio (step-length/step-rate). *Gait and Posture* **7**: 225–227.

Shiavi R. (1985) Electromyographic patterns in adult locomotion: a comprehensive review. *Journal of Rehabilitation Research and Development* **22**: 85–98.

Steindler A. (1953) A historical review of the studies and investigations made in relation to human gait. *Journal of Bone and Joint Surgery* **35A**: 540–542.

Sutherland DH. (1984) *Gait Disorders in Childhood and Adolescence*. Baltimore, MA: Williams & Wilkins.

Sutherland D. (1997) The development of mature gait. *Gait and Posture* **6**: 163–170.

Sutherland DH, Olshen RA, Biden EN, Wyatt MP. (1988) *The Development of Mature Walking*. London: MacKeith Press.

Todd FN, Lamoreux LW, Skinner SR *et al.* (1989) Variations in the gait of normal children. *Journal of Bone and Joint Surgery* **71A**: 196–204.

Wall JC, Charteris J, Turnbull GI. (1987) Two steps equals one stride equals what? The applicability of normal gait nomenclature to abnormal walking patterns. *Clinical Biomechanics* **2**: 119–125.

Waters RL, Mulroy S. (1999) The energy expenditure of normal and pathological gait. *Gait and Posture* **9**: 207–231.

Waters RL, Lunsford BR, Perry J, Byrd R. (1988) Energy–speed relationship of walking: standard tables. *Journal of Orthopaedic Research* **6**: 215–222.

Wells RP. (1981) The projection of the ground reaction force as a predictor of internal joint moments. *Bulletin of Prosthetic Research* **10(35)**: 15–19.

Winter DA. (1980) Overall principle of lower limb support during stance phase of gait. *Journal of Biomechanics* **13**: 923–927.

Winter DA. (1983) Energy generation and absorption at the ankle and knee during fast, natural, and slow cadences. *Clinical Orthopaedics and Related Research* **175**: 147–154.

Winter DA. (1991) *The Biomechanics and Motor Control of Human Gait*, 2nd edn. Waterloo, Ontario: University of Waterloo Press.

Winter DA. (1995) Human balance and posture control during standing and walking. *Gait and Posture* **3**: 193–214.

Winter DA, Quanbury AO, Reimer GD. (1976) Analysis of instantaneous energy of normal gait. *Journal of Biomechanics* **9**: 253–257.

3

Pathological and other abnormal gaits

Although some variability is present in normal gait, particularly in the use of the muscles, there is an identifiable 'normal pattern' of walking, and a 'normal range' can be defined for all of the measurable variables. Pathology of the locomotor system frequently produces gait patterns that are clearly 'abnormal'. Some of these abnormalities can be identified by eye, but others can only be identified by the use of appropriate measurement systems.

In order that a person can walk, the locomotor system must be able to accomplish four things:

1. Each leg in turn must be able to support the body weight without collapsing
2. Balance must be maintained, either statically or dynamically, during single leg stance
3. The swinging leg must be able to advance to a position where it can take over the supporting role
4. Sufficient power must be provided to make the necessary limb movements and to advance the trunk.

In normal walking, all of these are achieved without any apparent difficulty and with a modest energy consumption. However, in many forms of pathological gait they can be accomplished only by means of abnormal movements, which usually increase the energy consumption, or by the use of walking aids such as canes, crutches or orthotic devices (calipers and braces). If even one of these four requirements cannot be met, the subject is unable to walk.

The pattern of gait is the outcome of a complex interaction between the many neuromuscular and structural elements of the locomotor system. Abnormal gait may result from a disorder in any part of this system, including the brain, spinal cord, nerves, muscles, joints and skeleton. Abnormal gait may also result from the presence of pain, so that although a person is physically capable of walking normally, it may be more comfortable to walk in some other way.

The term 'limp' is commonly used to describe a wide variety of abnormal gait patterns. However, dictionary definitions are unhelpful, a typical one being 'to walk lamely'. Since the word has no clearly defined scientific meaning, it should only be used with caution in the context of gait analysis. The most appropriate use of the word is probably for a gait abnormality involving some degree of asymmetry that is readily apparent to an untrained observer.

Since gait is the end result of a complicated process, a number of different original problems may manifest themselves in the same abnormality of gait. For this reason, the abnormal gait patterns will be described separately from the pathological conditions that cause them. The first part of the chapter describes, in some detail, the commonest abnormal gait patterns. This is followed by a description of the use of walking aids, and the gait of amputees. The chapter ends with a description of the way in which gait abnormalities may result from a number of common but serious neurological conditions.

Specific gait abnormalities

The following section is based on a manual of lecture notes for student orthotists, published by New York University (1986). It includes a very useful list of common gait abnormalities, all of which can be identified by eye. The manual criticizes the common practice of identifying gait abnormalities by their pathological cause, for example 'hemiplegic gait', which immediately suggests that all hemiplegics walk in the same way. This is far from true, and also neglects the changes in gait that may occur with the passage of time, or as the result of treatment. The manual suggests that it is preferable to use purely descriptive terms, such as 'excessive medial foot contact'. This practice will be adopted in the following section. Some of the gait abnormalities described in the New York University publication applied only to the gait of subjects wearing orthotic devices; these descriptions have been omitted from the present text.

The pathological gait patterns to be described may occur either alone or in combination. If in combination they may interact, so that the individual gait modifications may not exactly fit the description. The list that follows is not exhaustive; a subject may use a variation of one of the general patterns, or may use another gait pattern that is not listed here.

When studying a pathological gait, particularly one that does not appear to fit into one of the standard patterns, it is helpful to remember that an abnormal movement may be performed for one of two reasons:

1. The subject has no choice, the movement being 'forced' on them by weakness, spasticity or deformity
2. The movement is a compensation, which the subject is using to correct for some other problem, which therefore needs to be identified.

Lateral trunk bending

Bending the trunk towards the side of the supporting limb during the stance phase is known as lateral trunk bending, ipsilateral lean or, more commonly, a *Trendelenburg gait*. The purpose of the maneuver is generally

Figure 3.1 Schematic of double-legged stance: the force in each hip joint (226 N) is half the weight of the trunk (452 N). The abductors are not contracting.

to reduce the forces in the abductor muscles and hip joint during single leg stance.

Lateral trunk bending is best observed from the front or the back. During the double support phase the trunk is generally upright, but as soon as the swing leg leaves the ground the trunk leans over towards the side of the stance phase leg, returning to the upright attitude again at the beginning of the next double support phase. The trunk bending may be unilateral, being restricted to the stance phase of one leg, or it may be bilateral, the trunk swaying from one side to the other, to produce a gait pattern known as *waddling*.

In the examples that follow, the weight of the trunk is 452 N, corresponding to a mass of 46 kg, and the weight of the right leg is 147 N, corresponding to a mass of 15 kg. As explained in Chapter 1, weight is a force, which is calculated by multiplying an object's mass by the acceleration due to gravity ($9.81 \, \text{m/s}^2$).

Fig. 3.1 shows a schematic of the trunk, pelvis and hip joints when standing on both legs. The abductor muscles are inactive, and the weight of the trunk is divided equally between the two hip joints. Fig. 3.2 shows what happens in a normal individual when the right foot is lifted off the ground: the force through the left hip joint increases by a factor of six, from 226 N (23 kgf or 51 lbf) to 1510 N (154 kgf or 339 lbf). This increase in force is made up of three components:

1. The whole of the weight of the trunk is now supported by the left hip joint, instead of being shared between the two hips
2. The weight of the right leg is now taken by the left hip, instead of by the ground
3. The left hip abductors (primarily gluteus medius) contract, producing an anticlockwise moment to keep the pelvis from dropping on the unsupported side. The reaction force to this contraction passes through the left hip.

These three components contribute to the increased force in the left hip as follows:

Figure 3.2 Schematic of single-legged stance. The force in the left hip (1510 N) is the sum of a) weight of trunk (452 N); b) weight of right leg (147 N), and c) contraction force of abductor muscles (911 N).

1. Trunk weight not shared:	226 N (23 kgf or 51 lbf)
2. Weight of right leg:	147 N (15 kgf or 33 lbf)
3. Contraction of abductors:	911 N (93 kgf or 204 lbf)
Total:	1284 N (131 kgf or 288 lbf)

It should be noted that this example was invented for the purposes of illustration – the actual numbers should not be taken too seriously!

The four conditions that must be met if this mechanism is to operate satisfactorily are:

1. The absence of significant pain on loading
2. Adequate power in the hip abductors
3. A sufficiently long lever arm for the hip abductors
4. A solid and stable fulcrum in or around the hip joint.

Should one or more of these conditions not be met, the subject may adopt lateral trunk bending in an attempt to compensate.

The effect of lateral trunk bending on the joint force is shown in Fig. 3.3. There is no effect on components (1) and (2) of the increased force, but if the center of gravity of the trunk is moved directly above the left hip, this eliminates the clockwise moment produced by the mass of the trunk. The abductors are now only required to contract with a force of 363 N (37 kgf or 81 lbf), to balance the clockwise moment provided by the weight of the right leg. There is thus a reduction of 548 N (56 kgf or 123 lbf) in the abductor contraction force, and a corresponding reduction in the total joint force, from 1501 N down to 962 N. The numbers in the illustrations refer to standing; during the stance phase of walking higher forces are to be expected due to the vertical accelerations of the center of gravity, which cause the force transmitted through the leg to fluctuate above and below body weight (Fig. 2.19). However, these fluctuations tend to be less in pathological than in normal gait, since the vertical accelerations are less in someone walking with a shorter stride length. The numbers also

Figure 3.3 Lateral trunk bending: bringing the trunk across the supporting hip reduces the clockwise moments about the left hip from 62 N·m to 25 N·m, permitting the pelvis to be stabilized by a smaller abductor force. The force in the left hip (962 N) is the sum of a) weight of trunk (452 N), b) weight of right leg (147 N), and c) contraction force of abductor muscles (363 N).

suppose that the bending of the trunk brings its center of gravity exactly above the hip joint. This is unlikely to happen in practice, of course, but the principles remain the same, whether the center of gravity is not deviated as far as the hip joint, or even if it passes lateral to it.

There are a number of conditions in which this gait abnormality is adopted:

1. *Painful hip*: if the hip joint is painful, as in osteoarthritis and rheumatoid arthritis, the amount of pain experienced usually depends to a very large extent on the force being transmitted through the joint. Since lateral trunk bending reduces the total joint force, Trendelenburg gait is extremely common in people with arthritis of the hip. Although it produces a useful reduction in force, and hence in pain, the forces still remain substantial (962 N in Fig. 3.3), and some form of definitive treatment is usually required.
2. *Hip abductor weakness*: if the hip abductors are weak, they may be unable to contract with sufficient force to stabilize the pelvis during single leg stance. In this case the pelvis will dip on the side of the foot that is off the ground (Trendelenburg's sign, as opposed to Trendelenburg gait). In order to reduce the demands on the weakened muscles the subject will usually employ lateral trunk bending, in both standing and walking, to reduce joint moment as far as possible (Fig. 3.4). Hip abductor weakness may be caused by disease or injury affecting either the muscles themselves or the nervous system that controls them.
3. *Abnormal hip joint*: three conditions around the hip joint will lead to difficulties in stabilizing the pelvis using the abductors: congenital dislocation of the hip (CDH, also known as developmental dysplasia of the hip), coxa vara and slipped femoral epiphysis. In all three the effective length of the gluteus medius is reduced because the greater trochanter of the femur moves upwards towards the pelvic brim. Since the muscle

Figure 3.4 Trendelenburg's sign: due to inadequate hip abductors: the pelvis drops on the unsupported side when one foot is lifted off the ground. To compensate, the subject bends the trunk over the supporting hip.

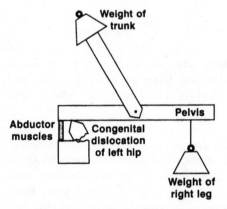

Figure 3.5 Congenital dislocation of the hip (CDH): both the working length and the lever arm of the hip abductors are reduced. To compensate, the subject bends the trunk over the supporting hip.

is shortened, it is unable to function efficiently, and thus contracts with a reduced tension. In CDH and severe cases of slipped femoral epiphysis a further problem exists, in that the normal hip joint is effectively lost, to be replaced by a false hip joint, or *pseudarthrosis*. This abnormal joint is more laterally placed, giving a reduced lever arm for the abductor muscles, and it may fail to provide the 'solid and stable fulcrum' mentioned above. The combination of reduced lever arm and reduced muscle force gives these subjects a powerful incentive to walk with lateral trunk bending (Fig. 3.5). In many cases, particularly in older people with CDH, the false hip joint becomes arthritic, and they add a painful hip to their other problems. Pain is frequently also a factor in slipped femoral epiphysis.

4. *Wide walking base*: if the walking base is abnormally wide, there is a problem with balance during single leg stance. Rather than tip the whole body to maintain balance, as in Fig. 2.27a, lateral bending of

the trunk may be used to keep the center of gravity of the body roughly over the supporting leg. In most cases this will need to be done during the stance phase on both sides, leading to bilateral trunk bending and a waddling gait. A wide walking base is a gait abnormality for which a number of causes exist, and these will be described later.

5. *Unequal leg length*: when walking with an unequal leg length, the pelvis tips downwards on the side of the shortened limb as the body weight is transferred to it. This is sometimes described as 'stepping into a hole'. The pelvic tilt is accompanied by a compensatory lateral bend of the trunk.

6. Other causes: Perry (1992) gives a number of other causes for lateral bending of the trunk, including adductor contracture, scoliosis, and an impaired body image, typically following a stroke.

Anterior trunk bending

In anterior trunk bending, the subject flexes his or her trunk forwards early in the stance phase. If only one leg is affected the trunk is straightened again around the time of opposite initial contact, but if both sides are affected the trunk may be kept flexed throughout the gait cycle. This gait abnormality is best seen from the side.

One important purpose of this gait pattern is to compensate for an inadequacy of the knee extensors. The left diagram of Fig. 3.6 shows that early in the stance phase, the line of action of the ground reaction force vector normally passes behind the axis of the knee joint and generates an external moment that attempts to flex it. This is opposed by contraction of the quadriceps, to generate an internal extension moment. If the quadriceps is weak or paralyzed it cannot generate this internal moment, and the knee will tend to collapse. As shown in the right-hand diagram of Fig. 3.6, anterior trunk bending is used to move the center of gravity of the body forwards, which results in the line of

Figure 3.6 Anterior trunk bending: in normal walking, the line of force early in the stance phase passes behind the knee; anterior trunk bending brings the line of force in front of the knee, to compensate for weak knee extensors.

force passing in front of the axis of the knee, producing an external extension (or hyperextension) moment. In addition to anterior trunk bending, subjects will sometimes keep one hand on the affected thigh while walking, to provide further stabilization for the knee.

Other causes for anterior trunk bending are equinus deformity of the foot, hip extensor weakness and hip flexion contracture (Perry, 1992).

Posterior trunk bending

One form of posterior trunk bending is essentially a reversed version of anterior trunk bending, in that early in the stance phase the whole trunk moves in the sagittal plane, but this time backwards instead of forwards. Again, it is most easily observed from the side. The purpose of this is to compensate for ineffective hip extensors. The line of the ground reaction force early in the stance phase normally passes in front of the hip joint (left diagram, Fig. 3.7). This produces an external moment which attempts to flex the trunk forward on the thigh, opposed by contraction of the hip extensors, particularly gluteus maximus. Should these muscles be weak or paralyzed, the subject may compensate by moving the trunk backwards at this time, bringing the line of action of the external force behind the axis of the hip joint as shown in the right-hand diagram of Fig. 3.7.

A different type of posterior trunk bending may occur early in the swing phase, where the subject may throw the trunk backwards in order to propel the swinging leg forwards. This is most often used to compensate for weakness of the hip flexors or spasticity of the hip extensors, either of which make it difficult to accelerate the femur forwards at the beginning of swing. This maneuver may also be used if the knee is unable to flex, since the whole leg must be accelerated forwards as one unit, which greatly

Normal   Posterior trunk bending

Figure 3.7 Posterior trunk bending: in normal walking, the line of force early in the stance phase passes in front of the hip; posterior trunk bending brings the line of force behind the hip, to compensate for weak hip extensors.

Increased lordosis

Figure 3.8 Increased lumbar lordosis: when there is a fixed flexion deformity of the hip (left), the whole pelvis must rotate forwards for the femur to move into a vertical position (right), with a resulting increase in lumbar lordosis.

increases the demands on the hip flexors. Posterior trunk bending may also occur when the hip is ankylosed (fused), the trunk moving backwards as the thigh moves forwards.

Increased lumbar lordosis

Many people have an exaggerated lumbar lordosis, but it is only regarded as a gait abnormality if the lordosis is used to aid walking in some way, which generally means that the degree of lordosis varies during the course of the gait cycle. Increased lumbar lordosis is best observed from the side of the subject, and generally reaches a peak at the end of the stance phase on the affected side.

The most common cause of increased lumbar lordosis is a flexion contracture of the hip. It is also seen if the hip joint is immobile due to ankylosis. Both of these deformities cause the stride length to be very short, by preventing the femur from moving backwards from its flexed position. This difficulty can be overcome if the femur can be brought into the vertical (or even extended) position, not through movement at the hip joint but by extension of the lumbar spine, with a consequent increase in the lumbar lordosis (Fig. 3.8).

The orientation of the pelvis in the sagittal plane is maintained by the opposing pulls of the trunk muscles above and the limb muscles below. If there is muscle imbalance – for example a weakness of the muscles of the anterior abdominal wall, weakness of the hip extensors or spasticity of the hip flexors – the subject may develop an excessive *anterior pelvic tilt*, again with an increase in the lumbar lordosis.

Functional leg length discrepancy

Four gait abnormalities (circumduction, hip hiking, steppage and vaulting) are closely related, in that they are designed to overcome the same problem – a functional discrepancy in leg length.

An 'anatomical' leg length discrepancy occurs when the legs are actually different lengths, as measured with a tape measure or, more accurately, by long-leg X-rays. A 'functional' leg length discrepancy means that the legs are not necessarily different lengths (although they may be), but that one or both are unable to adjust to the appropriate length for a particular phase of the gait cycle. In order for natural walking to occur, the stance phase leg needs to be longer than the swing phase leg. If it is not, the swinging leg collides with the ground and is unable to pass the stance leg. The way that a leg is functionally lengthened (for the stance phase) is to extend at the hip and knee and to plantarflex at the ankle. Conversely, the way in which a leg is functionally shortened (for the swing phase) is to flex at the hip and knee and to dorsiflex at the ankle. Failure to achieve all the necessary flexions and extensions is likely to lead to a functional leg discrepancy and hence to one of these gait abnormalities, which frequently occur as a result of a neurological problem. Spasticity of any of the extensors or weakness of any of the flexors tends to make a leg too long in the swing phase, as does the mechanical locking of a joint in extension. Conversely, spasticity of the flexors, weakness of the extensors, or a flexion contracture in a joint, makes the limb too short for the stance phase. Other causes of functional leg length discrepancy include musculoskeletal problems such as sacroiliac joint dysfunction.

An increase in functional leg length is particularly common following a stroke, where a foot drop (due to anterior tibial weakness or paralysis) may be accompanied by an increase in tone in the hip and knee extensor muscles.

The gait modifications designed to overcome the problem may either lengthen the stance phase leg or shorten the swing phase leg, thus allowing a normal swing to occur. They are not mutually exclusive, and a subject may use them in combination. The gait modification employed may have been forced on a particular person by the underlying pathology, or it may have been a matter of chance, two people with apparently identical clinical conditions having found different solutions to the problem.

Circumduction

Ground contact by the swinging leg can be avoided if it is swung outward, in a movement known as circumduction (Fig. 3.9). The swing phase of the other leg will usually be normal. The movement of circumduction is best seen from in front or behind.

Circumduction may also be used to advance the swinging leg in the presence of weak hip flexors, by improving the ability of the abductor muscles to act as hip flexors, while the hip joint is extended.

Hip hiking

Hip hiking is a gait modification in which the pelvis is lifted on the side of the swinging leg (Fig. 3.10) by contraction of the spinal muscles and the lateral abdominal wall. The movement is best seen from behind or in front.

By tipping the pelvis up on the side of the swinging leg, hip hiking involves a reversal of the second determinant of gait (pelvic obliquity about an antero-posterior axis). It may also involve an exaggeration of the first determinant (pelvic rotation about a vertical axis) to assist with

Figure 3.9 Circumduction: the swinging leg moves in an arc, rather than straight for-wards, to increase the ground clearance for the swing foot.

Figure 3.10 Hip hiking: the swing phase leg is lifted by raising the pelvis on that side.

leg advancement. Leg advancement may also be helped by posterior trunk bending at the beginning of the swing phase.

According to the manual by New York University (1986), hip hiking is commonly used in slow walking with weak hamstrings, since the knee tends to extend prematurely and thus to make the leg too long towards the end of the swing phase. It is seldom employed for limb lengthening due to plantarflexion of the ankle.

Steppage

Steppage is a very simple swing phase modification, consisting of exagger-ated knee and hip flexion, to lift the foot higher than usual for increased ground clearance (Fig. 3.11). It is best observed from the side.

Figure 3.11 Steppage: increased hip and knee flexion improve ground clearance for the swing phase leg, in this case necessitated by a foot drop.

Figure 3.12 Vaulting: the subject goes up on the toes of the stance phase leg to increase ground clearance for the swing phase leg.

It is particularly used to compensate for a plantarflexed ankle (commonly known as *foot drop*) due to inadequate dorsiflexion control, which will be described later.

Vaulting

The ground clearance for the swinging leg will be increased if the subject goes up on the toes of the stance phase leg, a movement known as vaulting (Fig. 3.12). This causes an exaggerated vertical movement of the trunk, which is both ungainly in appearance and wasteful of energy. It may be observed from either the side or the front.

Vaulting is a stance phase modification, whereas the related gait abnormalities (circumduction, hip hiking and steppage) are swing phase modifications. For this reason, vaulting may be a more appropriate solution for problems involving the swing phase leg. Like hip hiking, it is commonly used in slow walking with hamstring weakness, when the knee tends to extend too early in the swing phase. It may also be used on the 'normal' side of an above-knee amputee whose prosthetic knee fails to flex adequately in the swing phase.

Abnormal hip rotation

Because the hip is able to make large rotations in the transverse plane, for which the knee and ankle cannot compensate, an abnormal rotation at the hip involves the whole leg, with the foot showing an abnormal toe in or toe out alignment. The gait pattern may involve both stance and swing phases, and is best observed from behind or in front.

Abnormal hip rotation may result from one of three causes:

1. A problem with the muscles producing hip rotation
2. A fault in the way the foot makes contact with the ground
3. As a compensatory movement to overcome some other problem.

Problems with the muscles producing hip rotation usually involve spasticity or weakness of the muscles that rotate the femur about the hip joint. For example, overactivity of the hip extensors in cerebral palsy may include an element of internal rotation. Imbalance between the medial and lateral hamstrings is a common cause of rotation; weakness of biceps femoris or spasticity of the medial hamstrings will cause internal rotation of the leg. Conversely, spasticity of biceps femoris or weakness of the medial hamstrings will result in an external rotation.

A number of foot disorders will produce an abnormal rotation at the hip. Inversion of the foot, whether due to a fixed inversion (pes varus) or to weakness of the peroneal muscles, will internally rotate the whole limb when weight is taken on it. A corresponding eversion of the foot, whether fixed (pes valgus) or due to weakness of the anterior and posterior tibial muscles, will result in an external rotation of the leg.

External rotation may be used as a compensation for quadriceps weakness, to alter the direction of the line of force through the knee. This could be used as an alternative to, or in addition to, anterior trunk bending. External rotation may also be used to facilitate hip flexion, using the adductors as flexors if the true hip flexors are weak. Subjects with weakness of the triceps surae may externally rotate the leg to permit the use of the peroneal muscles as plantar flexors.

Excessive knee extension

In the gait abnormality of excessive knee extension the normal stance phase flexion of the knee is lost, to be replaced by full extension or even

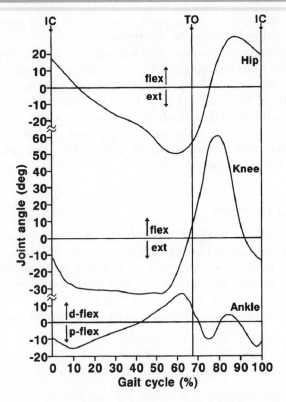

Figure 3.13 Excessive knee extension: sagittal plane hip, knee and ankle angles in a subject with paralyzed quadriceps, showing gross hyperextension of the knee and increased extension of the hip. Abbreviations as in Fig. 2.5.

hyperextension, in which the knee is angulated backwards. This is best seen from the side.

One cause of knee hyperextension has already been described: quadriceps weakness can be compensated for by keeping the leg fully extended, using anterior trunk bending (Fig. 3.6), external rotation of the leg, or both, to keep the line of the ground reaction force from passing behind the axis of the knee joint. Other means of keeping the knee fully extended are pushing the thigh back by keeping one hand on it while walking, and using the hip extensors to snap the thigh sharply back at the time of initial contact.

Hyperextension of the knee, accompanied by anterior trunk bending, is seen quite frequently in people with paralysis of the quadriceps following poliomyelitis. The gait abnormality is clearly of great value to the subject, since without it he or she would be unable to walk. However, the external hyperextension moment is resisted by tension in the posterior joint capsule, which gradually stretches, allowing the knee to develop a hyperextension deformity (genu recurvatum). As a result of this deformity, the joint frequently develops osteoarthritis in later life.

This is illustrated in Fig. 3.13, which shows the left sagittal plane hip, knee and ankle angles during walking in a 41-year-old woman whose quadriceps were paralyzed on both sides by poliomyelitis at the age of

12 years. She walked very slowly, using two forearm crutches (cycle time 1.9 s; cadence 63 steps/min; stride length 1.00 m; speed 0.52 m/s). The knee hyperextended to 32° during weight-bearing, but flexed normally to 63° during the swing phase. The hip extended more than in normal individuals, since hyperextension of the knee places the knee joint more posteriorly than usual, thus altering the angle of the femur.

In normal walking, an external moment attempts to hyperextend the knee during terminal stance. This is resisted by an internal flexor moment (Fig. 2.6), generated primarily by gastrocnemius. Should gastrocnemius be weak, the knee may be pushed backwards into hyperextension. This may help with walking, since the leg lengthening required during pre-swing can be provided by extending the knee rather than by plantarflexing the ankle. However, there is a risk that the knee will go beyond full extension into hyperextension, with consequent damage to the posterior capsule.

Hyperextension of the knee is common in spasticity. One common cause is overactivity of the quadriceps, which extends the knee directly. Another common cause is spasticity of the triceps surae, which plantarflexes the ankle and causes the body weight to be taken through the forefoot. The resulting forward displacement of the ground reaction force vector generates an external moment that is an exaggeration of the normal plantarflexion/knee extension couple, and results in hyperextension of the knee.

Shortness of one leg may cause a person, when standing, to take all his or her weight on the other (longer) leg, with the knee hyperextended. This is because it is uncomfortable to stand on both legs, since the knee on the longer side would have to be kept flexed.

Excessive knee flexion

The knee is normally fully extended (or nearly so) twice during the gait cycle – around initial contact and around heel rise. In the gait abnormality known as excessive knee flexion, one or both of these movements into extension fails to occur. The flexion and extension of the knee are best seen from the side of the subject.

A flexion contracture of the knee will obviously prevent it from extending normally. A flexion contracture of the hip may also prevent the knee from extending if hip flexion prevents the femur from becoming vertical or extended during the latter part of the stance phase (Fig. 3.14). By reducing the effective length of the leg during the stance phase, one of the compensations for a functional discrepancy in leg length will probably also be required.

Spasticity of the knee flexors may also cause the gait pattern of excessive knee flexion. Since the knee flexors are able to overpower the quadriceps, this may lead to other gait modifications, such as anterior trunk bending, to compensate for a relative weakness of the quadriceps.

The knee may flex excessively following initial contact if the normal plantarflexion of the foot during loading response is prevented through immobility of the ankle joint or a calcaneus deformity of the foot, thereby preventing the force vector from migrating forwards along the foot.

Figure 3.14 Excessive knee flexion: in late stance phase there is increased knee flexion, necessitated by a flexion contracture of the hip.

Increased flexion of the knee may also be part of a compensatory movement, either to reduce the effective limb length in functional leg length discrepancy, or as part of a pattern of exaggerated hip, knee and arm movements, to make up for a lack of plantarflexor power in push off.

Inadequate dorsiflexion control

The dorsiflexors are active at two different times during the gait cycle, so that inadequate dorsiflexion control may give rise to two different gait abnormalities. During loading response the dorsiflexors resist the external plantarflexion moment, thus permitting the foot to be lowered to the ground gently. If they are weak, the foot is lowered abruptly in a *foot slap*. The dorsiflexors are also active during the swing phase, when they are used to raise the foot and achieve ground clearance. Failure to raise the foot sufficiently during initial swing may cause *toe drag*. Both problems are best observed from the side of the subject, and both make a distinctive noise. Subjects with inadequate dorsiflexion control can often be diagnosed by ear, before they have come into view!

Inadequate dorsiflexion control may result from weakness or paralysis of the anterior tibial muscles, or from these muscles being overpowered by spasticity of the triceps surae. An inability to dorsiflex the foot during the swing phase causes a functional leg length discrepancy, for which a number of compensations were described previously. Toe drag will only be observed if the subject fails to compensate. Toe drag may also occur if there is delayed flexion of the hip or knee in initial swing, causing the foot to catch on the ground despite adequate dorsiflexion at the ankle.

Even if they suffer from inadequate dorsiflexion control, subjects with spasticity are frequently able to achieve dorsiflexion in the swing phase because flexion of the hip and knee are often accompanied by reflex

Figure 3.15 Talipes calcaneus.

Figure 3.16 Talipes equinus.

dorsiflexion of the ankle, in a primitive movement pattern related to the flexor withdrawal reflex mentioned in Chapter 1.

Abnormal foot contact

The foot may be abnormally loaded so that the weight is primarily borne on only one of its four quadrants. Loading on the heel or forefoot is best observed from the side, and loading on the medial or lateral side is best observed from the front, although some authorities state that the foot should always be observed from behind. Where a glass walkway is available, viewing the foot from below gives an excellent idea of the pattern of foot loading.

Loading of the heel occurs in the deformity known as *talipes calcaneus* (also known as pes calcaneus), where the forefoot is pulled up into extreme dorsiflexion (Fig. 3.15), usually as a result of muscle imbalance such as results from spasticity of the anterior tibial muscles or weakness of the triceps surae. Except in mild cases, weight is never taken by the forefoot, and the stance phase duration is reduced by the loss of the terminal rocker. The reduced stance phase duration on the affected side reduces the swing phase duration on the opposite side, which in turn reduces the opposite step length and the overall stride length. The ground reaction force vector remains posterior, producing an increased external flexion moment at the knee.

In the deformity known as *talipes equinus* (or pes equinus) (Fig. 3.16) the forefoot is fixed in plantarflexion, usually through spasticity of the plantar-flexors. In a mild equinus deformity the foot may be placed onto the ground flat; in more severe cases the heel never contacts the ground at all and initial contact is made by the metatarsal heads, in a gait pattern known as *primary toestrike*. Because the line of force from the ground

Figure 3.17 Talipes equinovarus.

reaction is displaced anteriorly, an increased external moment tending to extend the knee is present (plantarflexion/knee extension couple). The loss of the initial rocker shortens the stride length.

Excessive medial contact occurs in a number of foot deformities. Weakness of the inverters or spasticity of the everters will cause the medial side of the foot to drop and to take most of the weight. In *pes valgus*, the medial arch is lowered, permitting weight-bearing on the medial border of the foot. Increased medial foot contact may also be due to a valgus deformity of the knee, accompanied by an increased walking base.

Excessive lateral foot contact may also result from foot deformity, when the medial border of the foot is elevated or the lateral border depressed, by spasticity or weakness. The foot deformity known as *talipes equinovarus* (Fig. 3.17) combines equinus with varus, producing a curved foot where all the load is borne by the outer border of the forefoot. Although the term *club foot* may be applied to any foot deformity, it is most commonly applied to talipes equinovarus.

Another form of abnormal foot contact is the *stamping* that commonly accompanies a loss of sensation in the foot, such as occurs in tabes dorsalis, the final stage of syphilis. The subject receives feedback on ground contact from the vibration caused by the impact of the foot on the ground.

Abnormal foot rotation

Normal individuals place the foot on the ground approximately in line with the direction of walk, typically with a few degrees of toe out. Pathological toe in or toe out angles may be produced by internal or external hip rotation, torsion (twisting) of the femur or tibia, or deformity of the foot itself. An important consequence of an abnormal foot rotation is that it causes the ground reaction force to be in an abnormal position relative to the rest of the leg. For example, if the foot is internally rotated the ground reaction force is more medial than normal, which will generate external adductor moments at the ankle and knee. In either internal or external foot rotation, the length of the foot is reduced in the direction of progression, so that the ground reaction force during terminal stance and pre-swing is likely to be more posterior than normal. This reduces the lever arm for the triceps surae to generate an internal plantarflexion moment. This is one example of a problem known as *lever arm disease* or *lever arm deficiency*, in which individuals with normal muscle strength are unable to generate sufficient internal joint moments due to a reduction in the length of a muscle's lever arm. This is particularly seen in individuals with cerebral palsy who have a severe degree of internal or external foot rotation; the resulting posterior placement of the ground reaction force increases the external moment flexing the knee.

Insufficient push off

In normal walking, weight is borne on the forefoot during the push off in pre-swing. In the gait pattern known as insufficient push off, the weight is taken primarily on the heel and there is no push off phase, the whole foot being lifted off the ground at once. It is best observed from the side.

The main cause of insufficient push off is a problem with the triceps surae or Achilles tendon, which prevents adequate weight-bearing on the forefoot. Rupture of the Achilles tendon, or weakness of the soleus and gastrocnemius, are typical causes. Weakness or paralysis of the intrinsic muscles of the foot may also prevent the foot from taking load through the forefoot.

Insufficient push off may also result from any foot deformity, if the anatomy is so distorted that it prevents normal forefoot loading. A calcaneus deformity (Fig. 3.15) obviously makes it impossible to put any significant load on the forefoot.

Another important cause of insufficient push off is pain under the forefoot, if the amount of pain is affected by the degree of loading (as it usually is). This may occur in metatarsalgia, and also when arthritis affects the metatarsophalangeal joints. The loss of the terminal rocker causes the foot to leave the ground prematurely, before the hip has fully extended. This reduces the stance phase duration on the affected side, and hence the swing phase duration and step length on the opposite side, and produces an asymmetry in gait timing.

Abnormal walking base

The walking base is usually in the range of 50–130 mm. In pathological gait it may be either increased or decreased beyond this range. While ideally determined by actual measurement, changes in the walking base may be estimated by eye, preferably from behind the subject.

An increased walking base may be caused by any deformity, such as an abducted hip or valgus knee, which causes the feet to be placed on the ground wider apart than usual. A consequence of an increased walking base is that increased lateral movement of the trunk is required to maintain balance, as shown in Fig. 2.27.

The other important cause of an increased walking base is instability and a fear of falling, the feet being placed wide apart to increase the area of support. This allows a margin of error in the positioning of the center of gravity over the feet. This gait abnormality is likely to be present when there is a deficiency in the sensation or proprioception of the legs, so that the subject is not quite sure where the feet are, relative to the trunk. It is also used in cerebellar ataxia, to increase the level of security in an uncoordinated gait pattern. Another effective way to improve stability is to walk with one or two canes.

A narrow walking base usually results from an adduction deformity at the hip or a varus deformity at the knee. Hip adduction may cause the swing phase leg to cross the midline, in a gait pattern known as *scissoring*, which is commonly seen in cerebral palsy. In milder cases, the swing phase leg is able to pass the stance phase leg, but then moves across in front of it. In more severe cases, the swinging leg is unable to pass the stance leg: it stops behind it, with the side-to-side positions of the two feet reversed. This is clearly a very disabling gait pattern, with a very short stride length and negative values for the walking base and for the step length on one side.

Rhythmic disturbances

Gait disorders may include abnormalities in the timing of the gait cycle. Two types of rhythmic disturbance can be identified: an *asymmetric* rhythmic disturbance shows a difference in the gait timing between the two legs, and an *irregular* rhythmic disturbance shows differences between one stride and the next. Rhythmic disturbances are best observed from the side, and may also be audible.

An *antalgic* gait pattern is specifically a gait modification which reduces the amount of pain a person is experiencing. The term is usually applied to a rhythmic disturbance in which as short a time as possible is spent on the painful limb, and a correspondingly longer time is spent on the pain-free side. The pattern is asymmetrical between the two legs, but is generally regular from one cycle to the next. A marked difference in leg length between the two sides may also produce a regular gait asymmetry of this type, as may a number of other differences between the two sides, such as joint contractures or ankylosis.

Irregular gait rhythmic disturbances, where the timing alters from one step to the next, are seen in a number of neurological conditions. In particular, cerebellar ataxia leads to loss of the 'pattern generator', responsible for a regular, coordinated sequence of footsteps. Loss of sensation or proprioception may also cause an irregular arrhythmia, due to a general uncertainty about limb position and orientation.

Other gait abnormalities

A number of other gait abnormalities may be observed, either alone or in combination with some of the gait patterns described above. They include:

1. Abnormal movements, for example intention tremors and athetoid movements
2. Abnormal attitude or movements of the upper limb, including a failure to swing the arms
3. Abnormal attitude or movements of the head and neck
4. Sideways rotation of the foot following heelstrike
5. Rapid fatigue.

This account has concentrated on gait abnormalities that may be observed visually. However, a number of gait abnormalities can only be detected using kinetic/kinematic gait analysis systems. An example is the presence of an abnormal moment, such as the excessive internal varus moment that may be present in the knee of children with myelomeningocele and that may predispose them to the development of osteoarthritis (Lim *et al.*, 1998).

Walking aids

The use of walking aids may modify the gait pattern considerably. While some people use a walking aid to make it easier to walk, for example to reduce the pain in a painful joint, others are totally unable to walk without some form of aid. Although there are many detailed variations in design, walking aids, also called assistive devices, can be classified into three basic types – *canes*, *crutches* and *frames*. All three operate by supporting part of the body weight through the arm rather than the leg. While this is an effective way of coping with inadequacies of the legs, it frequently leads to problems with the wrist and shoulder joints, which are simply not designed for the transmission of large forces.

There is considerable variability in the way in which walking aids are used, and people will often use them in ways that do not quite fit the typical patterns described in the following sections.

Canes

The simplest form of walking aid is the cane, also known as a walking stick, by means of which force can be transmitted to the ground through the wrist and hand. Since the forearm muscles are relatively weak and the joints of the wrist fairly small, it is impossible to transmit large forces through a cane for any length of time. The torque that can be applied to the upper end of the cane is limited by the grip strength and by the shape of the handle, since the hand tends to slip. For this reason the major direction of force transmission is along the axis of the cane. Canes may be used for three purposes, which are often combined: to improve stability; to generate a moment; and to take part of the load away from one of the legs – i.e. to reduce limb loading.

1. *To improve stability*: Canes are frequently used by the elderly and infirm to improve their stability. This is achieved by increasing the size of the area of support, thus removing the need to position the center of gravity over the relatively small supporting area provided by the feet. In those with only minor stability problems, a single cane may be used. This will not provide a secure supporting area during single limb support, but does make it easier to correct for small imbalances. Since the cane is usually placed on the ground some distance away from the feet, giving a relatively long lever arm, a modest force through the cane will produce a substantial moment to correct for any positioning error. For maximum security a person will need to use two canes, so that a triangular supporting area is always available. This is provided by two canes and one foot during single limb support, and by one cane and two feet during double support. If only a single cane is used, it will

Figure 3.18 The use of a cane to generate a counterclockwise moment reduces the contraction force of the hip abductors, and hence the force in the hip joint. The force in the left hip (962 N) is the sum of a) weight of trunk (452 N); b) weight of right leg (147 N); c) contraction force of abductor muscles (463 N); less d) force through cane (100 N). (Compare with Fig. 3.2.)

normally be advanced during the stance phase of the more secure leg. If two canes are used, they are usually advanced separately, during double limb support, to provide the maximum stability at all times.

2. *To generate a moment:* The use of a cane to generate a moment is illustrated in Fig. 3.18. This should be compared with Fig. 3.2, which shows the mechanics of normal single-legged stance. A vertical force of 100 N (10 kgf or 22 lbf) is applied through the cane, which generates a counterclockwise moment, applied to the shoulder girdle and hence to the pelvis. This reduces the size of the moment that the hip abductor muscles need to generate to keep the pelvis level. The contraction of these muscles is reduced from 911 N (93 kgf or 204 lbf) to 463 N (47 kgf or 104 lbf), a reduction of 448 N (56 kgf or 123 lbf). The total force in the hip joint is reduced by the sum of this amount and the force applied by the cane to the ground. For this mechanism to work, the cane must be held in the opposite hand to the painful hip. A cane may also be used to generate a lateral moment at the knee, to reduce the loading on one side of the joint. The cane is advanced during the swing phase of the leg it is protecting.

3. *To reduce limb loading:* When using a cane to remove some of the load from the leg, it is usually held in the same hand as the affected leg and placed on the ground close to the foot. In this way load-sharing can be achieved between the leg and the cane, even to the extent of removing the load entirely from the leg. The cane follows the movements of the affected leg, being advanced during the swing phase on that side. The person will normally lean sideways over the cane, in a *lateral lurch*, to increase the vertical loading on it, and hence to reduce the load in the leg. A cane may be used in this way to relieve pain in the hip, knee,

ankle or foot. If the cane is held in the opposite hand, as is often recommended, the lateral lurching can be avoided, but the degree of off-loading is reduced.

Whichever of these three reasons a person has for using a cane, the degree of disability will determine whether one or two canes are used. It may be observed that a subject uses a cane in the opposite hand from that which might have been expected. In some cases he or she has simply not discovered that the benefits would be greater from using the cane in the other hand, but more often the observer has failed to appreciate fully all the compensations that the subject has adopted.

There are a number of ways in which the simple cane can be modified, including many different types of handgrip. A particularly important variant on the simple cane is the *broad-based cane*, also known as a *Hemi-* or *crab cane*, which may have three feet (*tripod*) or four feet (*tetrapod*, or *quad cane*). This differs from the simple cane in that it will stand up by itself, and will tolerate small horizontal force components, so long as the overall force vector remains within the area of its base. It is particularly helpful when standing up from the sitting position. The increased stability is gained at the expense of an increase in weight and particularly bulk, which may cause difficulties when going through doorways.

Crutches

The main difference in function between a crutch and a cane is that a crutch is able to transmit significant forces in the horizontal plane. This is because unlike the cane, which is effectively fixed to the body at only a single point, the crutch has two points of attachment (one at the hand and one higher up the arm), which provide a lever arm for the transmission of torque. Although there are many different designs of crutch, they fall into two categories – axillary crutches and forearm crutches. As with the cane, it is also possible to have a broad-based crutch, ending in three or four feet.

Axillary crutches (Fig. 3.19, left diagram), as their name suggests, fit under the axilla (armpit). They are usually of simple design, with a padded top surface and a handhold in the appropriate position. The lever arm between the axilla and the hand is fairly long, and enough horizontal force can be generated to permit walking when both legs are straight and non-functional. A disadvantage of this type of crutch is that the axilla is not an ideal area for weight-bearing, and incorrect fitting or prolonged use may cause damage to the blood vessels or nerves. Although some people use axillary crutches for many years they are more suitable for short-term use, for instance while a patient has a broken leg set in plaster.

There are many different types of *forearm crutches*, also called *elbow*, *Lofstrand* or *Canadian crutches* (Fig. 3.19, center diagram). They differ from axillary crutches in that the upper point of contact between the body and the crutch is provided by either the forearm or the upper arm, rather than by the axilla. The lever arm is thus shorter than for an axillary crutch, although this is seldom a problem, and they usually run less risk of tissue

Figure 3.19 Three types of crutch: axillary (left), forearm (center) and gutter (right).

damage, as well as being lighter and more acceptable cosmetically. In the normal forearm crutch most of the vertical force is transmitted through the hand, but the use of a 'gutter' or 'platform' permits more load to be taken by the forearm itself (Fig. 3.19, right diagram).

Walking frames

The most stable walking aid is the frame, also called a walker or Zimmer frame, which enables the subject to stand and walk within the area of support provided by its base. Considerable force can be applied to the frame vertically, and moderate forces can be applied horizontally, provided that the overall force vector remains within the area of support. The usual method of walking is first to move the frame forwards, then to take a short step with each foot, then to move the frame again, and so on. Walking is thus extremely slow, with a start–stop pattern. Although the subject is encouraged to lift the frame forward at each step, it is more often simply slid along the ground.

A *rollator* is a variant on the walking frame, in which the front feet are replaced by wheels. This makes it easier to advance, at the expense of a slight reduction in stability in the direction of progression. The mode of walking is very similar to that with the frame, except that it is easier to move forwards, since tipping the rollator lifts the back feet clear of the ground. Again, many subjects misuse the rollator by sliding it forwards rather than tipping it. A further variant on the design is to replace all four feet by wheels, which works well if effective brakes are provided. There are many other designs of frames and rollators, including ones that fold, and ones with 'gutters' to support the body weight through the forearms.

Figure 3.20 Four-point gait. One crutch or leg is moved at a time in the pattern left crutch – right leg – right crutch – left leg.

Gait patterns with walking aids

There are a number of different ways of walking when using a cane, crutch or walker. The terminology varies somewhat from one author to another; the descriptions that follow are based on the well-illustrated text by Pierson (1994). The first four gait patterns involve the greatest support from the upper limbs, by means of a walking frame, two crutches or two canes. The last two require less support, with a crutch or cane held in only one hand.

1. *Four-point gait* can be employed with canes or crutches. Also known as reciprocal gait, it involves the separate and alternate movement of each of the two legs and the two walking aids, for example: left crutch – right leg – right crutch – left leg (Fig. 3.20). This pattern is very stable and requires little energy, but it is very slow, so that the oxygen cost (oxygen consumption per unit distance) may be higher than for the three-point gait described below.
2. *Three-point gait* is used when only one leg can take weight, or the two legs move together as a single unit. It is only used with crutches or a walker. Two main forms of three-point gait are recognized – *step-through* and *step-to*. These terms are used when the lower limb musculature is able to provide the movement of the legs. If the legs are paralyzed, and their movement is provided by the upper limbs and trunk, the terms swing-through and swing-to are used (Pierson, 1994). In step-through gait, the foot or feet move from behind the line of the two crutches to in front of them (Fig. 3.21). This gait pattern requires a lot of energy and good control of balance, but it can be fairly fast. In step-to gait, the foot or feet are advanced to just behind the line of the crutches, which are then moved further forwards, and the process repeated (Fig. 3.22). Since the stride length is short, walking speed is low, but energy and stability requirements are not as high as for step-through gait.
3. *Modified three-point gait* (also known as *three–one gait*) may be used when one leg is able to take full body weight but the other is not. It may be employed with a walker, or with two crutches or canes. The walking aids and the affected leg move forward together, while weight is taken on the sound leg. That leg is then advanced, while weight is taken on

Figure 3.21 Three-point step-through gait in someone taking weight on both legs. The legs are advanced together, in front of the line of the crutches, then the crutches are advanced together, in front of the line of the legs.

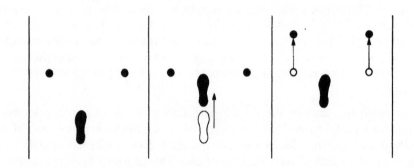

Figure 3.22 Three-point step-to gait in someone taking weight on only one leg. The leg is advanced to behind the line of the crutches, which are then moved forwards again.

the bad leg and the walking aids. This makes for a stable gait pattern, requiring little strength or energy, but the speed is fairly low.

4. *Two-point* gait resembles four-point gait, except that the crutch or cane on one side is moved forward at the same time as the leg on the other, for example: left crutch/right leg – right crutch/left leg. It is faster than four-point gait, yet is still fairly stable and requires little energy. However, it demands good coordination by the subject.

5. *Modified four-point gait* is performed when the walking aid is carried in the opposite hand to the affected leg. This gait pattern is typically used in hemiplegia, where there is paralysis of an arm and a leg on the same side. A typical walking sequence would be right crutch – left leg – right leg.

6. *Modified two-point gait* also involves the use of a walking aid on the opposite side to the bad leg, but the walking aid and the bad leg are moved forward together, for example: right crutch/left leg – right leg. It clearly needs better strength and coordination than modified four-point gait, but gives better speed.

Amputee gait

The majority of lower limb amputations are carried out at one of three levels: above knee (AK), below knee (BK), or at the level of the ankle (Syme's). Above knee and below knee amputations are often referred to as *transfemoral* and *transtibial* amputations, respectively. The degree of disability is significantly greater for AK amputees than for the other two groups. Nonetheless, people can adapt remarkably well to amputation, as demonstrated by those individuals who are able to run using an AK prosthesis.

Providing the amputation is carried out competently and the remaining muscles and nerves are normal, people with an AK amputation should have useful function in all the muscle groups acting about the hip joint. However, the mechanical coupling between the femur and the prosthetic limb can never be as good as in the normal individual, for three reasons:

1. The lever arm between the hip joint and the socket is relatively short, which reduces the moment that the hip muscles can apply to the prosthetic leg
2. There is always some relative motion between the stump of the femur and the socket due to the compression of soft tissues, which is exaggerated in the case of a poorly fitting socket
3. If the socket is uncomfortable, the subject may be reluctant to apply large forces to the prosthetic limb.

AK amputees lack any ability to resist an external flexion moment at the knee, and they must walk with the knee in full extension during single leg stance. They commonly use the gait modification of anterior trunk bending in order to keep the knee fully extended. In order to minimize the need for this gait modification, the flexion axis of prosthetic knee joints is normally placed more posterior than that of the natural knee, making it easier to keep the force vector in front of the joint. Walking with a stiff knee in the stance phase leads to greater rise and fall of the center of gravity than normal (loss of the third determinant of gait), and a consequent increase in energy expenditure. This type of walking is tiring, but nonetheless some people with one or even two AK amputations manage to get around extremely well. There have been some attempts to provide stance phase knee flexion, or its equivalent (shortening the leg through a telescopic action), but these devices have not yet come into widespread use.

Control of the knee joint in the swing phase is one of the most important requirements in the design of an AK prosthesis. If the knee joint is completely free, the pendulum action causes it to flex too quickly following toe off, so that the heel flicks up behind the subject. The knee then extends too rapidly, stopping abruptly as it hits the end stop in hyperextension. In contrast, a knee that permits no flexion or extension requires the whole leg to be accelerated and decelerated in one piece, which places enormous demands on the hip musculature and leads to much higher energy expenditure in walking (Saunders *et al.*, 1953). The compromise between these extremes is a prosthetic knee joint with some form of damping mechanism, which prevents all of these problems.

A variety of different damping mechanisms are available, including friction, hydraulic, pneumatic and computer-controlled systems. Murray *et al.* (1983) examined the gait of AK amputees using two different knee mechanisms, one of which gave a constant frictional load at all knee angles and one, using hydraulics, which varied its loading with knee angle and direction of motion. They found that the performance of the hydraulic mechanism was generally better. Amongst the differences they noted between normal and AK amputee gait, the duration of the swing phase was found to be longer on the amputated side, which resulted in an increased cycle time (decreased cadence). The stride length was close to normal, but the increased cycle time led to a decreased speed. Lateral trunk bending was often present; they attributed this partly to a compensation for a wider walking base, which was used to improve stability, and partly to a compensation for a decreased efficiency of the hip abductors due to movement of the femoral stump within the socket. Heel rise took place earlier in the stance phase than in normal individuals, because of a reduction in the ability to dorsiflex the prosthetic ankle. The magnitude of the heel rise in initial swing was increased, especially at higher walking speeds; it is very sensitive to the frictional properties of the knee mechanism. There was a tendency to vault on the normal leg during the swing phase of the prosthetic leg. Since the prosthetic leg shortened adequately during the swing phase, this vaulting was probably not necessary. It may have been used to gain added security, since the ground clearance of the prosthetic limb cannot be judged in the absence of proprioception. Unilateral amputees commonly show other abnormalities in the gait pattern of the sound limb.

Fig. 3.23 shows plots of the sagittal plane hip, knee and ankle angles in a 17-year-old female AK amputee with a hydraulic knee mechanism. It should be compared with Fig. 2.5, which shows comparable data from a normal subject. The knee moves into a few degrees of hyperextension well before the end of the swing phase, and remains hyperextended until pre-swing. The swing phase knee flexion is almost normal. The stance phase is a little shorter than normal. The hip movement is almost normal except for a sudden increase in flexion late in the swing phase, as the knee mechanism reaches its extension stop and the momentum of the swinging leg is transferred to the femur. Flexibility in the prosthetic foot leads to a fairly normal pattern of ankle motion, although the magnitudes of these movements are less than normal.

A below knee amputation deprives the user of the ability to plantarflex and dorsiflex the ankle, although the artificial foot normally provides some flexibility in this respect, and its shape provides partially functioning initial and terminal rockers. The loss of active plantarflexion at the end of the stance phase means that muscle power cannot be used to provide an active push off, and the effective length of the leg is shorter than normal, so that it has to be lifted clear of the ground sooner (Breakey, 1976). According to Saunders *et al.* (1953), the path of the center of gravity is essentially normal after a BK amputation, since the hip and knee together can largely compensate for the loss of the ankle joint. If both ankle and knee are lost, as in an AK amputation, the compensation is incomplete.

Fig. 3.24 shows the sagittal plane hip, knee and ankle angles of a

Figure 3.23 Sagittal plane hip, knee and ankle angles during walking in an above knee amputee. The main abnormality is hyperextension of the knee, from before initial contact to just before toe off. Abbreviations as in Fig. 2.5.

Figure 3.24 Sagittal plane hip, knee and ankle angles during walking in a below knee amputee. The ankle angle shows slight abnormalities. Abbreviations as in Fig. 2.5.

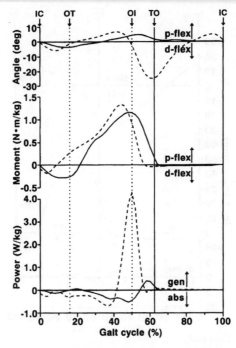

Figure 3.25 Sagittal plane ankle angle, internal moment and power in a below knee amputee (solid line) and normal subject (dashed line). Abbreviations as in Figs 2.5–2.7.

47-year-old male BK amputee using a 'multiflex' foot, walking with a cycle time of 1.26 s (cadence 95 steps/min), stride length 1.45 m and speed 1.15 m/s, all of which are towards the lower end of the normal range. The hip and knee angles are within normal limits. The ankle angle is also nearly normal, although the movement into plantarflexion at the end of the stance phase is of relatively low magnitude and occurs a little late. This is because it is a passive movement, resulting from the removal of loading from the elastic foot mechanism rather than the active plantarflexion seen in normal subjects.

Fig. 3.25 shows the sagittal plane angle, moment and power from the prosthetic ankle of a 35-year-old male BK amputee using a SACH foot (solid ankle, cushion heel) prosthesis, walking with a cycle time of 1.13 s (cadence 106 steps/min), stride length 1.54 m and speed 1.37 m/s. The corresponding records from the normal subject used for illustration in Chapter 2 are shown as dashed lines. The ankle range of motion during the gait cycle in this subject was very restricted, with no plantarflexion around toe off. The ankle moment shows that the prosthesis attempted to retain a fairly neutral position, resisting plantarflexion during the loading response and resisting dorsiflexion during mid-stance and terminal stance. As a result, little power exchange took place until terminal stance, when the ankle absorbed a little power in becoming maximally dorsiflexed. Part of this was returned in power generation as the moment reduced, and the ankle returned towards the neutral position. However, the power generation involved was very small when compared with the normal individual.

Other designs of prosthetic foot are better able to store and return energy, and research continues in this area.

As can be seen from Figs 3.24 and 3.25, there are considerable differences between subjects in amputee gait. Neither pattern corresponded particularly well to the description by Breakey (1976) of the 'typical' gait pattern of the BK amputee:

1. Delayed foot flat
2. Reduced stance phase knee flexion
3. Early heel rise
4. Early toe off
5. Reduced stance phase duration
6. Reduced swing phase knee flexion.

Treadmill gait

It is often more convenient to study gait while the subject walks on a treadmill rather than over the ground, since the volume in which measurements need to be made is much smaller and they can conveniently be connected to wires or breathing tubes. However, there are subtle differences between treadmill and overground gait, particularly with regard to joint angles. The reduced airflow over the body is unlikely to be a significant factor, but the subject's awareness of the limited length of the treadmill belt may cause shortening of the stride length. However, the most important differences are probably due to changes in the speed of the treadmill belt as the subject's feet decelerate it at initial contact and accelerate it at push off, effectively storing energy in the treadmill motor. This effect is minimized by using a large treadmill with a powerful motor (Savelberg *et al.*, 1998).

Common pathologies affecting gait

While many pathological conditions can cause an abnormal gait, a group of neurological conditions stand out as being particularly important. If the basic defect is in the brain, the gait abnormality is often very complex, and accurate diagnosis may only be possible using the techniques of systematic gait analysis. In contrast, gait abnormalities due to more peripheral disorders, such as diseases of the joints, tend to be much easier to identify and interpret. The following sections outline the gait disorders that may result from some relatively common conditions that affect the brain.

Cerebral palsy

The assessment of patients with cerebral palsy (CP) is one of the most important applications of gait analysis (Õunpuu *et al.*, 1996).

Cerebral palsy usually follows brain damage around the time of birth. It involves a loss of the selective control of muscles by the motor cortex, and the emergence of spasticity and primitive patterns of contraction. As a general rule the muscles are not weak, but they may be unable to contract adequately at appropriate times in the gait cycle due to a loss of coordination. Muscular contraction cannot be turned on or off rapidly, and there is commonly a co-contraction of antagonists. Similar deficits are often seen in children or adults who have suffered traumatic brain injury.

The characteristics of CP were given by Gage (1991) as follows:

1. Loss of selective muscle control
2. Dependence on primitive reflex patterns for ambulation
3. Abnormal muscle tone
4. Relative imbalance between muscle agonists and antagonists across joints
5. Deficient equilibrium reactions.

There is considerable variation between one patient and another in the way in which CP affects the positions and movements of the joints. The clinical picture depends on which muscles are affected, and on the timing of their contraction during the gait cycle.

Many patients with cerebral palsy are incapable of walking. The majority of those who are able to walk have either spastic hemiplegia or spastic diplegia. Since this condition is so variable, deciding what combination of treatments is best for a particular patient can be extremely difficult. This application is one of the most important uses for clinical gait analysis, as will be discussed further in Chapter 5. Strictly speaking, hemiplegia implies a total paralysis on one side of the body, and hemiparesis a partial paralysis, although the word 'hemiplegia' is often applied loosely to both conditions.

Spastic hemiplegia

Spastic hemiplegia is the commonest neurological cause of an abnormal gait. As well as occurring in cerebral palsy, it is also frequently seen in elderly people who have suffered a cerebrovascular accident ('stroke'). It may also occur following traumatic brain injury. The characteristics of hemiparetic gait following a stroke were reviewed by Olney and Richards (1996). A companion paper (Richards and Olney, 1996) reviewed the natural history and treatment of the condition. Hemiplegic gait is characterized by spasticity and loss of function in some or all of the muscles of one side of the body, the other side being normal or nearly normal. The arms are usually affected more than the legs, and patients with hemiplegia generally walk with the affected arm held immobile, in a characteristic flexed posture. A hemiplegic patient usually possesses a mixture of normal motor control, spasticity and patterned responses, the exact combination depending on the severity and location of the brain damage (Perry, 1969). As well as the problems they experience with moving and controlling their limbs, many hemiplegic patients also have problems in maintaining balance, because a defect in the 'body image' causes them to ignore the affected side.

Since only one side of the body is affected, the majority of people with spastic hemiplegia are able to walk. Winters *et al.* (1987) showed that the gait pattern of children and young adults with this condition could be divided into four groups. These are numbered I to IV in order of increasing severity, each group having all the neurological deficits of the preceding one with some additions. In general, the results of this study of young people agreed with other publications on the gait of elderly subjects who had suffered a cerebrovascular accident. Gage (1991) gave a very clear, illustrated account of this classification. Subsequent studies have confirmed the validity of this classification and provided information on the differences between the groups in terms of moments, powers and energy consumption.

Group I subjects essentially suffer from a single problem – a foot drop on the affected side. This causes initial contact to be by primary toestrike, and also produces a functional increase in leg length during the swing phase. According to Winters *et al.* (1987), the plantarflexed attitude of the foot at initial contact results in several compensations: increased flexion of the knee and hip ('steppage'), and an increased lumbar lordosis. The most common surgical treatment for this problem is to lengthen the Achilles tendon. However, this is unlikely to improve the gait, since the ankle is usually able to dorsiflex adequately. The significant problem in these individuals is the foot drop during the swing phase, caused by a relative weakness of the anterior tibial muscles, which can be treated adequately by a simple ankle–foot orthosis (AFO).

Group II subjects, as well as having a foot drop, have a static or dynamic contracture of the calf muscles, which holds the ankle in plantarflexion throughout the whole of the gait cycle. The difference in gait between Group I and Group II subjects is seen after mid-stance, when the persistent plantarflexion produces an external moment which forces the knee into hyperextension (the plantarflexion/knee extension couple). According to Winters *et al.* (1987), advancement of the trunk is curtailed and the length of the opposite step is decreased. As with the Group I subjects, there is increased hip flexion with an associated increased lumbar lordosis. These patients generally benefit from an operation to lengthen the Achilles tendon, as well as an orthosis to control the foot drop.

Group III subjects have a foot drop, contracted calf muscles, and over-activity of both quadriceps and hamstrings. This causes a reduction in the total range of motion at the knee, with a marked reduction in swing phase flexion and a consequent increase in functional leg length. Since the opposite leg is usually fairly normal, many of these patients respond by vaulting on the sound side (Gage, 1991). The other features of the Group II pattern are also present: hyperextension of the knee in late stance, hip flexion and increased lumbar lordosis. Surgical correction of these patients will extend as high as the knee. Waters *et al.* (1979) showed that the stiff-legged gait is caused by an inappropriate contraction of one or more heads of the quadriceps (especially rectus femoris), during pre-swing and initial swing. Gage (1991) recommended hamstrings lengthening, combined with transfer of the rectus femoris so that it acts as a knee flexor rather than an extensor.

The greatest degree of neurological involvement is seen in Group IV subjects. In addition to the characteristics of the Group III subjects, they also have a reduced range of hip motion due to overactivity of iliopsoas and the adductors. The hip is unable to extend fully, so anterior pelvic tilt and increased lumbar lordosis at the end of the stance phase are used to preserve the stride length. Full treatment of these patients includes lengthening the hip flexors (primarily psoas major), in addition to surgery to the muscles acting about the knee and ankle joints.

Spastic diplegia

Spastic diplegia is a common manifestation of cerebral palsy. It primarily affects the legs, although there may be considerable asymmetry between the two sides. According to Gage (1991), most individuals with spastic diplegia are of normal intelligence. As its name suggests, spasticity is a particularly prominent element of this condition. The tension in the spastic muscles during development often leads to bony deformities, especially a torsion, or twisting, of the femur (femoral anteversion) and the tibia (external tibial torsion). A further significant problem in spastic diplegia is often a lack of stability in standing and walking. Many individuals with this condition continue to need walking aids, even after surgical treatment, to correct for deficiencies in balance.

There are considerable variations between individuals, but the commonest pattern consists of:

1. Hip flexion and internal rotation, due to overactivity by the iliopsoas, rectus femoris and hip adductors
2. Knee flexion, due to overactivity of the hamstrings, especially on the medial side
3. Equinus deformity of the foot and eversion of the hindfoot, due to overactivity by the triceps surae and peronei.

Excessive flexion of the hips leads to an increased lumbar lordosis, in order to get the femur as vertical as possible (Fig. 3.8). The knee is held almost fixed by co-contraction of the hamstrings and quadriceps. Since the hamstrings are the more powerful of the two muscle groups, the knee remains flexed, and its angle typically varies only between 30 and 40° of flexion. The equinus deformity of the foot causes a primary toestrike, and loss of all three 'rockers' – plantarflexion in loading response, dorsiflexion in mid-stance and plantarflexion in pre-swing.

The hip, knee and ankle angles on the left side of a 6-year-old girl with spastic diplegia are shown in Fig. 3.26 (adapted from Gage, 1983). The hip angle, defined here as the angle between the femur and vertical, was fairly normal, although the pelvis was tilted forwards to compensate for tight hip flexors. The knee never extended beyond 25° of flexion, due to overactivity of the hamstrings. The plantarflexed position of the ankle throughout the cycle is evident, initial contact being made by the forefoot rather than the heel, because of spasticity of the triceps surae. Particularly striking on this plot is the very long stance phase and very short swing phase.

One difficulty in managing spastic diplegia is in determining the causes of inappropriate joint angles. For example, excessive hip flexion may be due to overactive hip flexors, or it may be due to the anterior knee position caused by increased knee flexion – or both! Similarly, initial contact by the forefoot,

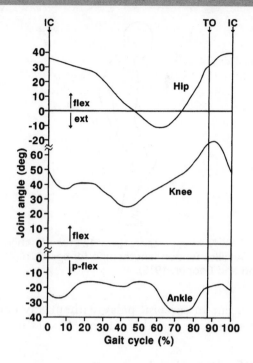

Figure 3.26 Sagittal plane hip, knee and ankle angles during walking in the left leg of a 6-year-old girl with spastic diplegia (adapted from Gage, 1983). Abbreviations as in Fig. 2.5.

rather than the heel, may be due to a static or dynamic ankle plantarflexion, or again it may be the result of the altered geometry caused by walking with a flexed knee. The functional leg length inequality caused by a lack of swing phase knee flexion commonly leads to a coping response, such as circumduction, hip hiking or vaulting. It is the aim of systematic gait analysis to determine the causes of the observed gait abnormalities, and to use this information as the basis for planning treatment.

The pattern described above is not the only one seen in spastic diplegia, which is a highly variable condition. Significant numbers of patients walk with hyperextension of the knee and a stiff-legged gait, which interferes with foot clearance during the swing phase.

An occasional complication of the treatment of cerebral palsy is the development of a *crouch gait* (Fig. 3.27), which may occur spontaneously (see below), but is particularly likely if an equinus deformity of the foot is over-corrected, in the presence of a flexion contracture of the knee (Sutherland and Cooper, 1978). Excessive lengthening of the Achilles tendon may be caused directly by surgery, or it may be caused by post-operative stretching. The result is a calcaneus deformity of the foot, which keeps the line of the ground reaction force a long way behind the already flexed knee. This leads to a vicious circle in which the increased external moment leads to an increased force in the quadriceps, which gradually stretches the patellar tendon, further increasing the knee flexion and hence the external moment. Sutherland and Cooper (1978) stressed the need to correct the knee deformity before operating on the heel cord.

Figure 3.27 Position of body at mid-stance in a 12-year-old child with crouch gait, following Achilles tendon lengthening for spastic diplegia (adapted from Sutherland and Cooper, 1978).

Crouch gait may occur in cerebral palsy without any operative intervention, as a result of spasticity of either the hip flexors or the hamstrings.

Other varieties of cerebral palsy

The detailed classification of cerebral palsy is a complicated subject, which will only be touched on here, but which has been well described by Gage (1991). As far as the clinical use of gait analysis is concerned, the most important categories are spastic hemiplegia and spastic diplegia, described above. *Spastic quadriplegia* affects all four limbs, the legs worse than the arms. Those who are affected by it are seldom able to walk, except in its milder forms, when the problems and approaches to treatment are similar to those described for spastic diplegia. Occasionally a patient is seen who has all four limbs affected, but the arms are worse than the legs. This condition is sometimes known as *double hemiplegia*. The other major category in the classification of cerebral palsy involves the extrapyramidal system, and includes abnormalities of movement such as *athetosis* in which one or more limbs are 'waved about' in a seemingly random manner. Patients with such conditions can seldom be helped by the use of gait analysis or the types of treatment discussed above (Gage, 1991).

Myelomeningocele

Myelomeningocele (often loosely referred to as spina bifida) results from a failure of the lower part of the spinal cord to develop normally. Depending largely on how much of the spinal cord is affected, the neurological deficit may range from negligible to extensive. Many individuals with this condition are able to walk, and gait analysis is often used for assessment and planning treatment (Õunpuu *et al.*, 1996).

Vankoski *et al.* (1995) divided children with the mildest (lumbosacral) form of myelomeningocele into three groups on the basis of plantarflexor muscle strength, group II being the most affected, group IB being intermediate, and group IA the least affected. Group IA patients could generally walk without the use of an ankle–foot orthosis (AFO). The plantarflexor strength generally correlated with the strength of other muscle groups, especially the hip extensors. The authors illustrated the patterns of motion of the pelvis, hip and knee for individuals in all three groups, with and without AFOs.

Parkinsonism

The condition known as parkinsonism (also known as Parkinson's disease) is a disorder of the extrapyramidal system, caused by degeneration of the basal ganglia of the brain. Amongst its other clinical features it includes a *shuffling gait*. Murray *et al.* (1978) examined the gait of 44 men with parkinsonism, and identified the following abnormalities:

1. Stride length and speed were very much reduced, although cycle time was usually normal
2. The walking base was slightly increased
3. The range of motion at the hip, knee and ankle were all decreased, mainly by a reduction in joint extension
4. The swinging of the arms was much reduced
5. The majority of patients rotated the trunk in phase with the pelvis, instead of twisting it in the opposite direction
6. The vertical trajectories of the head, heel and toe were all reduced, although other workers have commented on a distinct 'bobbing' motion of the head.

The 'shuffle' occurred because the foot was still moving forward at the time of initial foot contact. In some patients initial contact was made by the flat foot; in others there was a heelstrike, but the foot was much more horizontal than usual. Some patients also showed scuffing of the foot in mid-swing. Unlike most gait patterns, which stabilize within the first two or three steps, the gait of patients with parkinsonism often 'evolves' over the course of several strides.

Other conditions

As was mentioned previously, many different conditions affect gait, only a few of which have been described in detail. Cerebral palsy and parkinsonism were singled out for a more detailed discussion, since they can be extremely complicated, and often lead to combinations of different gait deviations. The effects of these and other conditions will be further considered in Chapter 5, which deals with the practical application of the methods of gait analysis.

References and suggestions for further reading

Breakey J. (1976) Gait of unilateral below-knee amputees. *Orthotics and Prosthetics* **30**: 17–24.

Gage JR. (1983) Gait analysis for decision-making in cerebral palsy. *Bulletin of the Hospital for Joint Diseases Orthopaedic Institute* **43**: 147–163.

Gage JR. (1991) *Gait Analysis in Cerebral Palsy.* London: MacKeith Press.

Lim R, Dias L, Vankoski S et al. (1998) Valgus knee stress in lumbosacral myelomeningocele: a gait-analysis evaluation. *Journal of Pediatric Orthopaedics* **18**: 428–433.

Murray MP, Sepic SB, Gardner GM, Downs WJ. (1978) Walking patterns of men with parkinsonism. *American Journal of Physical Medicine* **57**: 278–294.

Murray MP, Mollinger LA, Sepic SB et al. (1983) Gait patterns in above-knee amputee patients: hydraulic swing control vs constant-friction knee components. *Archives of Physical Medicine and Rehabilitation* **64**: 339–345.

New York University (1986) *Lower Limb Orthotics.* New York: Prosthetics and Orthotics, New York University Postgraduate Medical School.

Olney SJ, Richards C. (1996). Hemiparetic gait following stroke. Part I: characteristics. *Gait and Posture* **4**: 136–148.

Õunpuu S, Davis RB, DeLuca PA. (1996) Joint kinetics: methods, interpretation and treatment decision-making in children with cerebral palsy and myelomeningocele. *Gait and Posture* **4**: 62–78.

Perry J. (1969) The mechanics of walking in hemiplegia. *Clinical Orthopaedics and Related Research* **63**: 23–31.

Perry J. (1990) Pathologic gait. *American Academy of Orthopaedic Surgeons: Instructional Course Lectures* **39**: 325–331.

Perry J. (1992) *Gait Analysis: Normal and Pathological Function.* Thorofare, NJ: SLACK Incorporated.

Pierson FM. (1994) *Principles and Techniques of Patient Care.* Philadelphia, PA: W.B. Saunders Co.

Richards CL, Olney SJ. (1996) Hemiparetic gait following stroke. Part II: recovery and physical therapy. *Gait and Posture* **4**: 149–162.

Saunders JBDM, Inman VT, Eberhart HS. (1953) The major determinants in normal and pathological gait. *Journal of Bone and Joint Surgery* **35A**: 543–558.

Savelberg HHCM, Vorstenbosch MATM, Kamman EH et al. (1998) Intra-stride belt-speed variation affects treadmill locomotion. *Gait and Posture* **7**: 26–34.

Sutherland DH, Cooper L. (1978) The pathomechanics of progressive crouch gait in spastic diplegia. *Orthopedic Clinics of North America* **9**: 143–154.

Sutherland DH. (1984) *Gait Disorders in Childhood and Adolescence.* Baltimore: Williams & Wilkins.

Vankoski SJ, Sarwark JF, Moore C, Dias L. (1995) Characteristic pelvic, hip, and knee kinematic patterns in children with lumbosacral myelomeningocele. *Gait and Posture* **3**: 51–57.

Waters RL, Garland DE, Perry J et al. (1979) Stiff-legged gait in hemiplegia: surgical correction. *Journal of Bone and Joint Surgery* **61A**: 927–933.

Winters TF, Gage JR, Hicks R. (1987) Gait patterns in spastic hemiplegia in children and young adults. *Journal of Bone and Joint Surgery* **69A**: 437–441.

4

Methods of gait analysis

Gait analysis is used for two very different purposes: to aid directly in the treatment of individual patients, and to improve our understanding of gait through research. Gait research use may be further subdivided into 'fundamental' studies of walking, and clinical research. These topics are explored further in the next chapter. Clearly no single method of analysis is suitable for such a wide range of uses, and a number of different methodologies have been developed.

When considering the methods that may be used to perform gait analysis, it is useful to regard them as being in a spectrum or continuum, ranging from the absence of technological aids at one extreme to the use of complicated and expensive equipment at the other. This chapter starts with a method that requires no equipment at all, and goes on to describe progressively more elaborate systems. As a general rule, the more elaborate the system, the higher the cost, but the better the quality of objective data that can be provided. However, this does not imply that some of the simpler techniques are not worth using. It has often been found, particularly in a clinical setting, that the use of high technology gait analysis is inappropriate because of its high cost in terms of money, space and time, and because the clinical problem can be adequately managed using simpler techniques.

Visual gait analysis

It is tempting to say that the simplest form of gait analysis is that made by the unaided human eye. This, of course, neglects the remarkable abilities of the human brain to process the data received by the eye. Visual gait analysis is, in reality, the most complicated and versatile form of analysis available. Despite this, it suffers from four serious limitations:

1. It is transitory, giving no permanent record
2. The eye cannot observe high-speed events
3. It is only possible to observe movements, not forces
4. It depends entirely on the skill of the individual observer.

Table 4.1 Common gait abnormalities and best direction for observation

Gait abnormality	Observing direction
Lateral trunk bending	Side
Anterior trunk bending	Side
Posterior trunk bending	Side
Increased lumbar lordosis	Side
Circumduction	Front or behind
Hip hiking	Front or behind
Steppage	Side
Vaulting	Side or front
Abnormal hip rotation	Front or behind
Excessive knee extension	Side
Excessive knee flexion	Side
Inadequate dorsiflexion control	Side
Abnormal foot contact	Front or behind
Abnormal foot rotation	Front or behind
Insufficient push off	Side
Abnormal walking base	Front or behind
Rhythmic disturbances	Side

In a study on the reproducibility of visual gait analysis, Krebs *et al.* (1985) found it to be 'only moderately reliable'. Saleh and Murdoch (1985) compared the performance of people skilled in visual gait analysis with the data provided by a combined kinetic/kinematic system. They found that the measurement system identified many more gait abnormalities than had been seen by the observers.

Many clinicians include the observation of a subject's gait as part of their clinical examination. However, this is not gait analysis if it is limited to watching the subject make a single walk up and down the room. This merely gives a superficial idea of how well the subject walks, and perhaps identifies the most serious abnormality. A thorough visual gait analysis, as recommended in the manual from New York University (1986), involves watching the subject while he or she makes a number of walks, some of which are observed from one side, some from the other side, some from the front and some from the back. As the subject walks, the observer should look for the presence or absence of a number of specific gait abnormalities, such as those described in Chapter 3 and summarized in Table 4.1. A logical order should be used for looking for the different gait abnormalities – the mixture of walking directions listed in the table is not recommended! According to Rose (1983), it is also important when performing visual gait analysis to compare the range of motion at the joints during walking with those that are observed on the examination plinth – they may be either more or less.

The minimum length required for a gait analysis walkway is a hotly debated subject. The author believes that 8 m (26 ft) is about the minimum for use with fit young people, but that 10–12 m (33–39 ft) is preferable, since it permits fast walkers to 'get into their stride' before any measurements are made. However, shorter walkways are satisfactory for people who walk more slowly. This particularly applies to those with a

Front view camera

10 m

Line of walk

6 m

4 m

Side view camera

Distance mark on floor

Figure 4.1 Layout of a small gait laboratory for visual gait analysis, videotaping and measurement of the general gait parameters.

pathological gait, since the gait pattern usually stabilizes within the first two or three steps. A notable exception to this, however, is the gait in parkinsonism, which 'evolves' over the first few strides. The width required for a walkway depends on what equipment, if any, is being used to make measurements. For visual gait analysis, as little as 3 m (10 ft) may be sufficient. If videotape is being used, the camera needs to be positioned a little further from the subject, and about 4 m (13 ft) is needed. A kinematic system making simultaneous measurements from both sides of the body normally requires a width of at least 5–6 m (16–20 ft). Fig. 4.1 shows the layout of a small gait laboratory used for visual gait analysis, videotape and the measurement of the general gait parameters.

Some investigators permit subjects to choose their own walking speed, whereas others control the cycle time (or cadence), for example by asking them to walk in time with a metronome. The rationale for controlling the cycle time is that many of the measurable parameters of gait vary with the walking speed, and using a controlled cycle time provides one means of reducing the variability. However, subjects are unlikely to walk naturally when trying to keep pace with a metronome, and patients with motor control problems may find it difficult or even impossible to walk at an imposed cycle time. Zijlstra *et al.* (1995) found considerable differences in the gait of normal subjects between 'natural' walking and 'constrained' walking, in which the subject was required either to step in time with a metronome or to step on particular places on the ground. The answer to this dilemma is probably to accept the fact that subjects need to walk at different speeds, and to interpret the data appropriately. This means that 'normal' values must be available for a range of walking speeds. An unresolved difficulty with this approach is that it may not be possible to get 'normal' values for very slow walking speeds, since normal individuals do not customarily walk very slowly, and when asked to do so, some of the gait measurements become very variable (Brandstater *et al.*, 1983).

Gait assessment

Simply observing the gait and noting abnormalities is of little value by itself. It needs to be followed by gait assessment, which is the synthesis of these observations with other information about the subject obtained from the history and physical examination, combined with the intelligence and experience of the observer (Rose, 1983). Visual gait analysis is entirely subjective, and the quality of the analysis depends on the skill of the person performing it. It can be an interesting exercise to perform visual gait analysis on people walking past in the street, but without knowing their clinical details it is easy to misinterpret what is wrong with them.

One thing that must be constantly borne in mind when performing any type of gait analysis is that you are observing effects and not causes. Putting it another way, the observed gait pattern is not the direct result of a pathological process, but the net result of a pathological process and the subject's attempts to compensate for it. The observed gait pattern is 'what is left after the available mechanisms for compensation have been exhausted' (Rose, 1983).

Videotape examination

The widespread use of videotape has provided one of the most useful enhancements to gait analysis during recent years. It helps to overcome two of the limitations of visual gait analysis – the lack of a permanent record and the difficulty of observing high-speed events. In addition, it confers the following advantages:

1. It reduces the number of walks a subject needs to do
2. It makes it possible to show the subject exactly how they are walking
3. It makes it easier to teach visual gait analysis to someone else.

Videotape analysis is not an objective method, since it does not provide quantitative data in the form of numbers. However, it does provide a permanent record, which can be extremely valuable. The presence of an earlier videotape of a subject's gait may be used to demonstrate to all concerned how much progress has been made, especially when this has occurred over a long period of time. In particular, it may convince the subject and family members that an improvement *has* occurred, when memory tells them that things are no better than they were several months ago!

The most practical system consists of a camera-recorder (camcorder) to do the videotaping, and a separate videocassette recorder (VCR) to replay the tapes. The majority of today's domestic camcorders are perfectly suitable for use in gait analysis, the requirements being a zoom lens, automatic focus, the ability to operate in normal room lighting, and an electronically shuttered charge-coupled device (CCD) sensor to eliminate blurring due to movement. The VCR used to view the tapes should have a rock-steady freeze-frame facility, without any 'stripes' across the picture, and the ability to single-step successive frames, either one at a time or at a very slow speed. Such features are now available on many domestic VCRs, making them perfectly suitable for use in a clinical gait laboratory.

Videotape may thus be used to visualize events that are too fast for the unaided eye. For convenience, the camcorder should use the same size cassette as the VCR that will be used to view the tapes, thus avoiding the need for tape copying. Many gait laboratories now record video data directly into a computer, and this may be synchronized with data collection on a kinematic system (described later).

In making a thorough visual gait analysis without the use of videotape, the subject needs to make repeated walks to confirm or refute the presence of each of the gait abnormalities listed in Table 4.1. If the subject is in pain or easily fatigued, this may be an unreasonable requirement, and it may be difficult to achieve a satisfactory analysis. The use of videotape permits the subject to do a much smaller number of walks, as the person performing the analysis can rewind the tape and watch it as many times as necessary.

Videotape facilitates the process of teaching visual gait analysis, in which the student often needs to see small abnormal movements that happen very quickly. It is much easier to see such movements if the gait can be examined in slow motion, with the instructor pointing out details on the television monitor. The use of videotape also makes it possible to observe a variety of abnormal gaits that have been archived on tape. A number of teaching videotapes are now available (Appendix 3).

Showing a subject a videotape of his or her own gait is not exactly biofeedback, since there is a time delay involved, but nonetheless it can be very helpful. When a therapist is working with a subject to correct a gait abnormality, the subject may gain a clearer idea of exactly what the therapist is concerned about if it is possible to observe his or her own gait from the 'outside'.

Although visual gait analysis using videotape is subjective, it is easy, at the same time, to derive some objective data – the general gait parameters (cycle time or cadence, stride length and speed). The method will be described in the next section. It is also possible to measure joint angles, either directly from the monitor screen, or using some form of on-screen digitizer. Such measurements tend to be fairly inaccurate, however, because the limb may not be viewed from the correct angle, and because of distortions introduced by the television camera, the VCR and (especially) the television display.

Individual investigators will find their own ways of performing gait analysis using videotape, but the author's own routine may prove useful as a starting point. Subjects are asked to wear shorts or a swimsuit, so that the majority of the leg is visible. It is important that subjects should walk as normally as possible, so they are asked to wear their own indoor or outdoor shoes, with socks if preferred. Unless it would unduly tire them, it is a good idea for subjects to make one or two 'practice' walks before starting videotaping. The camera position, or the zoom lens, is first adjusted to show the whole body from head to feet, and subjects are videotaped from the side as they walk the length of the walkway in one direction. At the end they turn around, with a rest if necessary, and are videotaped as they walk back again. The whole process is then repeated, with the camera adjusted to show a close-up of the body from the waist down. Then either the camera position is changed or the subjects are asked to walk along a different pathway, so that they can be videotaped while walking away from the camera and then back towards it again. Two walks in each direction are again videotaped, although the magnification does not need to be changed, since this view automatically provides a range of views from close-up to full-body.

It is often helpful to mark the subjects' skin, for example using an eyebrow pencil, to enhance the visibility of anatomical landmarks on videotape. Hillman *et al.* (1998) fitted subjects with surface-mounted rotation indicators, to improve the accuracy with which transverse plane rotations can be estimated from videotape.

Subjects should not be able to see themselves on a monitor while they are walking, as this provides a distraction, particularly for children. Whether they are shown the videotape afterwards is at the discretion of the investigator, although it is important to review the tape before subjects leave, in case the recording needs to be repeated for some reason.

The analysis is performed by replaying the videotape, looking for specific gait abnormalities in the different views, and interpreting what is seen in the light of the subject's history and physical examination. It is particularly helpful if two or more people work together to perform the analysis. Rose (1983) suggested that gait analysis should be based on the team approach, with discussion and hypothesis testing. As will be described in Chapter 5, hypothesis testing may involve an attempted modification of the gait – for instance by fitting an orthosis, or by paralyzing a muscle using local anaesthetic.

General gait parameters

The general gait parameters (also known as the temporal and distance factors of gait) are the cycle time (or cadence), stride length and speed. These provide the simplest form of objective gait evaluation (Robinson and Smidt, 1981). Although there are automatic ways of making these measurements, which will be described in the next section, they may also be made using only a stopwatch, a tape measure and (optionally) some talcum powder. The method described below under 'General gait parameters from videotape' enables the simultaneous measurement of all three of the general gait parameters. It does not in fact require the patient's gait to be recorded on videotape, since it can be used while the patient's gait is being observed.

Cycle time, stride length and speed tend to change together in most locomotor disabilities, so that a subject with a long cycle time will usually also have a short stride length and a low speed (speed being stride length divided by cycle time). The general gait parameters give a guide to the walking ability of a subject, but little specific information. They should always be interpreted in terms of the expected values for the subject's age and sex, such as those given in Appendix 1. Fig. 4.2 shows one way in which these data may be presented; the diamonds represent the 95 per cent confidence limits for a normal subject of the same age and sex as the subject under investigation. Although cycle time is gradually replacing cadence in the gait analysis community, it is more

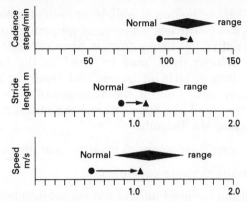

Figure 4.2 Display of the general gait parameters, with normal ranges appropriate for a patient's age and sex. Pre- and postoperative values for a 70-year-old female patient undergoing knee replacement surgery.

convenient to use cadence on plots of this type, since an abnormally slow gait will give values on the left-hand side of the graph for all three of the general gait parameters.

Cycle time or cadence

Cycle time or cadence may be measured with the aid of a stopwatch, by counting the number of individual steps taken during a known period of time. It is seldom practical to count for a full minute, so a period of 10 or 15 seconds is usually chosen. The loss of accuracy incurred by counting for such short periods of time is unlikely to be of any practical significance. Subjects should be told to walk naturally, and they should be allowed to get up to their full walking speed before the observer starts to count the steps. The cycle time is calculated using the formula:

$$\text{Cycle time (s)} = \text{time (s)} \times 2/\text{steps counted}$$

The number 2 allows for the fact that there are two steps per stride. The cadence is calculated using the formula:

$$\text{Cadence (steps/min)} = \text{steps counted} \times 60/\text{time (s)}$$

The number 60 allows for the fact that there are 60 seconds in a minute.

Stride length

Stride length can be determined in two ways – by direct measurement, or indirectly from the speed and cycle time. The simplest direct method of measurement is to count the strides taken while the subject covers a known distance. A more useful method (but a rather messy one!) is to have the subject step with both feet in a shallow tray of talcum powder, and then walk across a polished floor or along a strip of brown paper or colored construction paper, leaving a trail of footprints. These may be measured, as shown in Fig. 2.3, to derive left and right step lengths, stride length, walking base, toe-out angle, and some idea of the foot contact pattern. This investigation is able to provide a great deal of useful information, for the sake of a few minutes of mopping up the floor afterwards! As an alternative to using talcum powder, felt adhesive pads, soaked in different colored dyes, may be fixed to the feet (Rose 1983). The subject walks along a strip of paper, and leaves a pattern of dots, which give an accurate indication of the locations of both feet.

If both the cycle time and the speed have been measured, stride length may be calculated using the formula:

$$\text{Stride length (m)} = \text{speed (m/s)} \times \text{cycle time (s)}$$

The equivalent calculation using cadence is:

$$\text{Stride length (m)} = \text{speed (m/s)} \times 2 \times 60/\text{cadence (steps/min)}$$

The multiplication by 2 converts steps to strides, and by 60 converts minutes to seconds. For accurate results, the cycle time and speed should be measured during the same walk. However, the simultaneous counting, measuring and timing may prove to be too difficult, and the errors introduced by using data from different walks are not likely to be important unless the subject's gait varies markedly from one walk to another.

Speed

The speed may be measured by timing subjects while they walk a known distance, for example between two marks on the floor or between two pillars in a corridor. The distance walked is a matter of convenience, but somewhere in the region of 6–10 m (20–33 ft) is probably adequate. Again, subjects should be told to walk at their natural speed, and they should be allowed to get into their stride before the measurement starts. The speed is calculated as follows:

$$\text{Speed (m/s)} = \text{distance (m)/time (s)}$$

General gait parameters from videotape

Determination of the general gait parameters from a videotape of the subject walking is easy, providing the tape shows the subject passing two landmarks whose positions are known. One simple method is have the subject walk across two lines on the floor, a known distance apart, made with adhesive tape. Space should be allowed for acceleration before the first line, and for slowing down after the second one. When the videotape is played, the time taken to cover the distance is measured, and the steps taken are counted. It is easiest to take the first initial contact *beyond the start line* as the point to begin both timing and counting, and the first initial contact *beyond the finish line* as the point to end both timing and counting. This is not strictly accurate from a measurement point of view, but the errors introduced are likely to be trivial. As mentioned above, this method can also be used without videotaping the patient.

Since the distance, the time and the number of steps are all known, the general gait parameters can be calculated using the formulae:

$$\text{Cycle time (s)} = \text{time (s)} \times 2/\text{steps counted}$$

$$\text{Cadence (steps/min)} = \text{steps counted} \times 60/\text{time (s)}$$

$$\text{Stride length (m)} = \text{distance (m)} \times 2/\text{steps counted}$$

$$\text{Speed (m/s)} = \text{distance (m)}/\text{time (s)}$$

Timing the gait cycle

A number of systems have been described which perform the automatic measurement of the timing of the gait cycle, sometimes called the temporal gait parameters. Such systems may be divided into two main classes – footswitches and instrumented walkways. Fig. 4.3 shows typical data, which could be obtained from either type of system.

Footswitches

Footswitches are used to record the timing of gait. If one switch is fixed beneath the heel and one beneath the forefoot, it is possible to measure the timing of initial contact, foot flat, heel rise and toe off, and the duration of the stance phase (Figs 2.2 and 4.3). Data from two or more strides make it possible to calculate cycle time and swing phase duration. If switches are mounted on both feet, the single and double support times can also be measured. The footswitches are usually connected through a trailing wire to a computer, although alternatively either a radio transmitter or a portable recording device may be used to collect the data and transfer them to the measuring equipment.

Figure 4.3 Output from footswitches under the heel, four metatarsals (MT 1 to MT 4) and hallux of both feet. The switch is 'on' (i.e. the area is in contact with the ground) when the line is high.

A footswitch is exposed to very high forces, which may cause problems with reliability. This has led to many different designs being tried over the years. A fairly reliable footswitch may be made from two layers of metal mesh, separated by a thin sheet of plastic foam with a hole in it. When pressure is applied, the sheets of mesh contact each other through the hole and complete an electrical circuit. Footswitches are most conveniently used with shoes, although suitably designed ones may be taped directly beneath the foot. Small switches may also be mounted in an insole and worn inside the shoe. In addition to the basic heel and forefoot switches, further switches may be used in other areas of the foot to give greater detail on the temporal patterns of loading and unloading. In addition to the home-made varieties, a number of companies also manufacture footswitches.

Instrumented walkways

An instrumented walkway is used to measure the timing of foot contact, the position of the foot on the ground, or both. Many different designs have been developed, usually individually built for a single laboratory. The descriptions that follow refer to typical designs rather than to any particular system.

A conductive walkway is a gait analysis walkway that is covered with an electrically conductive substance, such as sheet metal, metal mesh or conductive rubber. Suitably positioned electrical contacts on the subject's shoes complete an electrical circuit. The conductive walkway is thus a slightly different method of implementing footswitches, and provides essentially the same information. Again, the subject usually trails an electrical cable, which connects the foot contacts to a computer. The speed needs to be determined independently, typically by having the body of the subject interrupt the beams of two photoelectric cells, one at each end of the walkway, again connected to the computer. Timing information from the foot contacts is used to calculate the cycle time, and the combination of cycle time and speed may be used to calculate the stride length.

An alternative arrangement is to have the walkway itself contain a large number of switch contacts, which detect the position of the foot as well as the timing of heel contact and toe off. This has the advantage that no trailing wires are required, and the walkway can be used to measure both step lengths and the stride length. A number of commercial systems are available to make this type of measurement, often also providing some information on the magnitude of the forces between the foot and the ground.

Direct motion measurement systems

A number of systems have been described which measure the motion of the body or legs, using some form of direct connection to the subject. As a general rule, direct measurement systems are more likely to be found in research laboratories than in clinical settings, and they are gradually giving way to other methods of measurement.

The simplest of these systems measures the forward displacement of the trunk by means of a light string, which is connected to the back of a belt around the subject's waist. As the individual walks forwards, the string is pulled through an instrument that measures its motion. This may be achieved in a number of ways, including a tacho-generator, which is a form of dynamo, the output voltage of which relates to the instantaneous speed of the string; or a device such as an optical encoder, which can be used to measure the length of the string as it passes through. Such systems will give the mean speed of walking, and also the instantaneous speed as it changes during the gait cycle.

A more elaborate system, based on the same principle, may be used to measure pelvic twist about the vertical axis by having one string attached to each side of the waist. It is also possible to measure lateral displacement in walking by having one or two strings running sideways, although some means must be provided to cope with the forward motion, such as by having the subject walk on a treadmill.

Direct connection systems may also be used to measure the motion of the legs. One such system uses perforated paper tape attached to the heels of both shoes, which is pulled through an optical reader as the subject walks forwards (Law, 1987; Law and Minns, 1989). This gives timing and displacement information for both feet, enabling the calculation of the cycle time, the two step lengths, stride length, speed, stance and swing phase durations, and the two double support times. Another system, which gives similar information, is based on a small trolley that is towed along behind the subject by a loop of cord, the ends of which are attached to the two feet (Klenerman *et al.*, 1988). The cord runs backwards and forwards through a measuring instrument on the trolley, and its movements provide the temporal and distance parameters of gait. The designers of both systems claimed that the subject is not aware of any drag produced by the attachments to the feet.

Electrogoniometers

An electrogoniometer is a device for making continuous measurements of the angle of a joint. The output of an electrogoniometer is usually plotted as a chart of joint angle against time, as shown in Fig. 2.5. However, if measurements have been made from two joints (typically the hip and the knee), the data may be plotted as an *angle–angle diagram*, also known as a cyclogram, shown in Fig. 4.4. This format makes clearer the interaction between the two joints, and makes it possible to identify characteristic patterns.

Potentiometer devices

A rotary potentiometer is a variable resistor, of the type used as a radio volume control, in which turning the central spindle produces a change in

Figure 4.4 Angle–angle diagram of the sagittal plane hip angle (horizontal axis) and knee angle (vertical axis). Initial contact is at the lower right. Normal subject; same data as Fig. 2.6.

electrical resistance that can be measured by an external circuit. It can be used to measure the angle of a joint if it is fixed in such a way that the body of the potentiometer is attached to one limb segment and the spindle to the other. The electrical output thus depends on the joint position, and the device can be calibrated to measure the joint angle in degrees. Many laboratories have constructed their own electrogoniometers of this type, and there have in the past been a few commercially available designs.

Although any joint motion could be measured by an electrogoniometer, they are most commonly used for the knee and less commonly for the ankle and hip. Fixation is usually achieved by cuffs, which wrap around the limb segment above and below the joint. The position of the potentiometer is adjusted to be as close to the joint axis as possible. A single potentiometer will only make measurements in one axis of the joint, but two or three may be mounted in different planes to make multi-axial measurements (Fig. 4.5). Trailing wires are normally used to connect the potentiometers to the measuring equipment, which is usually a computer.

Concern has been expressed about the accuracy of measurement provided by these potentiometer devices, since they are subject to a number of possible types of error, described below.

1. The electrogoniometer is fixed by cuffs around the soft tissues, not to the bones, so that the output of the potentiometer does not exactly relate to the true bone-on-bone movement at the joint.
2. Some designs of electrogoniometer will only give a true measurement of joint motion if the potentiometer axis is aligned to the anatomical axis of the joint. This may not be achievable for three reasons:
   a) it may be difficult to identify the joint axis, e.g. because of the depth of the hip joint below the surface
   b) the joint axis may not be fixed, e.g. the polycentric flexion–extension axis of the knee
   c) the rotation axis may be inaccessible, e.g. the internal–external rotation axis of the knee.
3. A joint may, in theory, move with up to six degrees of freedom – that is, it may have angular motion about three mutually perpendicular axes,

Figure 4.5 Subject wearing triaxial goniometers on hip, knee and ankle. Adapted from manufacturer's literature (Chattecx Corporation).

and linear motion ('translations') in three directions. In practice, the linear motion is usually negligible, particularly at the hip and ankle, and most electrogoniometer systems simply 'lose' any motion that does occur, either through the elasticity of the mounting cuffs or through a sliding or parallelogram mechanical linkage. However, where the electrogoniometer axis does not correspond exactly with the anatomical axis, larger linear motions will occur.

4. The output of the device gives a relative angle rather than an absolute one, and it may be difficult to decide what limb angle should be taken as zero, particularly in the presence of a fixed deformity.

Because of these problems, electrogoniometers are more p clinical setting (in which great accuracy is not usually neec the scientific laboratory. Chao (1980) addressed some of the in a defense of the use of potentiometer-based electrogoniome analysis.

Figure 4.6 Subject wearing flexible goniometers on knee and ankle. Adapted from manufacturer's literature (Biometrics Ltd).

Flexible strain gauges

The flexible strain gauge electrogoniometer (Fig. 4.6), manufactured by Biometrics Ltd (Cwmfelinfach, Gwent, UK), consists of a flat, thin strip of metal, one end of which is fixed to the limb on each side of the joint being studied. The bending of the metal as the joint moves is measured by strain gauges and their associated electronics. Because of the way in which metal strips respond to bending, the output depends simply on the angle between the two ends, linear motion being ignored. To measure motion in more than one axis a two-axis goniometer may be used, or two or three separate goniometers may be fixed around the joint, aligned to different planes.

Other electrogoniometers

With the increasing use of television-based kinematic systems (see below), electrogoniometers are declining in popularity. Other designs that have been used in the past include mercury-in-rubber, in which the electrical resistance of a column of mercury in an elastic tube changes as the tube is stretched across a joint, and an optical system known as the polarized light goniometer.

Pressure beneath the foot

The measurement of the pressure beneath the foot is a specialized form of gait analysis, which may be of particular value in those conditions (such as diabetic neuropathy and rheumatoid arthritis) in which the pressure may be excessive. Lord *et al.* (1986) reviewed a number of such systems. Foot pressure measurement systems may be either floor-mounted or in the form of an insole within the shoe.

The SI unit for pressure is the pascal (Pa), which is a pressure of one newton per square meter. The pascal is inconveniently small, and practical measurements are made in kilopascals (kPa) or megapascals (MPa).

Conversions between different units of measurement will be found in Appendix 2.

Lord *et al.* (1986) pointed out that when making measurements beneath the feet it is important to distinguish between force and pressure (force per unit area). Some of the measurement systems measure the force (or 'load') over a known area, from which the mean pressure over that area can be calculated. However, the mean pressure may be much lower than the peak pressure within the area if high pressure-gradients are present, which are often caused by subcutaneous bony prominences such as the metatarsal heads.

A pitfall which must be borne in mind when making pressure measurements beneath the feet is that a subject will normally avoid walking on a painful area. Thus, an area of the foot that had previously experienced a high pressure and become painful may show a low pressure when it is tested. However, this will not happen if the sole of the foot is anesthetic, as commonly occurs in diabetic neuropathy. In this condition, very high pressures, leading to ulceration, may be recorded.

Typical pressures beneath the foot are 80–100 kPa in standing, 200–500 kPa in walking, and up to 1500 kPa in some sporting activities. In diabetic neuropathy, pressures as high as 1000–3000 kPa have been recorded. To put these figures into perspective, the normal systolic blood pressure, measured at the feet in the standing position, is below 33 kPa (250 mm Hg); applied pressures that are higher than this will prevent blood from reaching the tissues.

Glass plate examination

Some useful semi-quantitative information on the pressure beneath the foot can be obtained by having the subject stand on, or walk across, a glass plate, which is viewed from below with the aid of a mirror or television camera. It is easy to see which areas of the sole of the foot come into contact with the walking surface, and the blanching of the skin gives an idea of the applied pressure. Inspection of both the inside and the outside of a subject's shoe will also provide useful information about the way the foot is used in walking – it is a good idea to ask patients to wear their oldest shoes when they come for an examination, not their newest ones!

Direct pressure mapping systems

A number of low-technology methods of estimating pressure beneath the foot have been described over the years. The Harris or Harris-Beath mat is made of thin rubber, the upper surface of which consists of a pattern of ridges of different heights. Before use it is coated with printing ink and covered by a sheet of paper, after which the subject is asked to walk across it. The highest ridges compress under relatively light pressures, the lower ones requiring progressively greater pressures, making the transfer of ink to the paper greater in the areas of the highest pressure. This gives a semi-quantitative map of the pressure distribution beneath the foot. Other systems have also been described in which the subject walks

Figure 4.7 Pressure beneath a cavus foot on landing from a jump (E.M. Hennig, 5th
Biennial Conference, Canadian Society of Biomechanics, 1988).

on a pressure-sensitive film, a sheet of aluminum foil, or something like a
typist's carbon paper.

Pedobarograph

The pedobarograph uses an elastic mat laid on top of an edge-lit glass
plate. When the subject walks on the mat it is compressed onto the glass,
which loses its reflectivity, becoming progressively darker with increasing
pressure. This darkening provides the means for quantitative measurement.
The underside of the glass plate is usually viewed by a television camera,
the monochrome image being processed to give a false-color display, in
which different colors correspond to different levels of pressure.

Force sensor systems

A number of systems have been described in which the subject walks
across an array of force sensors, each of which measures the vertical
force beneath a particular area of the foot. Dividing the force by the area
of the cell gives the mean pressure beneath the foot in that area. Many
different types of force sensor have been used, including resistive and
capacitative strain gauges, conductive rubber, piezoelectric materials, and
a photo-elastic optical system. A number of different methods have been
used to display the output of such systems, including the attractive presentation shown in Fig. 4.7.

In-shoe devices

The problem of measuring the pressure inside the shoe has been tackled in
a number of centers. The main difficulties with this type of measurement

are the curvature of the surface, a lack of space for the transducers, and the need to run large numbers of wires from inside the shoe to the measuring equipment. Nonetheless, a number of commercial systems are now available, which may give clinically useful results. Details of such systems may be found on the Internet (Appendix 3).

Electromyography

Electromyography (EMG) is the measurement of the electrical activity of a contracting muscle – the muscle action potential. Since it is a measure of electrical and not mechanical activity, the EMG cannot be used to distinguish between concentric, isometric and eccentric contractions, and the relationship between EMG activity and the force of contraction is far from straightforward. One of the most useful textbooks on the EMG is that by Basmajian (1974). The use of the EMG in the biomechanical analysis of movement was reviewed by Kleissen *et al.* (1998).

The three methods of recording the EMG are by means of surface, fine-wire and needle electrodes. In gait analysis EMG is usually measured with the subject walking, as opposed to the semi-static EMG measurements that are often made for neurological diagnosis.

Surface electrodes

Surface electrodes are fixed to the skin over the muscle, the EMG being recorded as the voltage difference between two electrodes. It is usually necessary also to have a grounding electrode, either nearby or elsewhere on the body. Since the muscle action potential reaches the electrodes through the intervening layers of fascia, fat and skin, the voltage of the signal is relatively small, and it is usually amplified close to the electrodes, using a very small pre-amplifier. The EMG signal picked up by surface electrodes is the sum of the muscle action potentials from many motor units within the most superficial muscle or muscles. Most of the signal comes from within 25 mm of the skin surface, so this type of recording is not suitable for deep muscles such as the iliopsoas. The EMG data may not be very specific, even with superficial muscles, due to interference from adjacent muscles ('crosstalk'). It is safest to regard the signal from surface electrodes as being derived from muscle groups rather than from individual muscles, although Õunpuu *et al.* (1997) showed that surface electrodes could satisfactorily distinguish between the three superficial muscle bellies of the quadriceps in children. There is often a change in the electrical baseline as the subject moves ('movement artifact'), and there may also be electromagnetic interference, for example from nearby electrical equipment.

Fine-wire electrodes

Fine-wire electrodes are introduced directly into a muscle, using a hypodermic needle, which is then withdrawn, leaving the wires in place. They can be quite uncomfortable or even painful. The wire is insulated, except for a few millimeters at the tip. The EMG signal may be recorded in three different ways:

1. Between a pair of wires inserted using a single needle
2. Between two fine wires, inserted separately
3. Between a single fine-wire and a ground electrode.

The voltage recorded within the muscle is generally higher than that from surface electrodes, particularly if separate wires are used, and there is less interference from movement and from electromagnetic fields. The signal is derived from a fairly small region of a single muscle, generally from a few motor units, a fact that must be taken into account when interpreting the data. Because it is an uncomfortable and invasive technique, fine-wire EMG is usually only performed on selected muscles and in patients in whom it is likely to be particularly useful.

Needle electrodes

Needle electrodes are generally more appropriate to physiological research than to gait analysis. A hypodermic needle is used, which contains an insulated central conductor. This records the EMG signal from a very local area within the muscle into which it is inserted, normally recording signals from only a single motor unit.

Limitations of EMG

The main problem with the use of any form of EMG is that it is at best only a semi-quantitative technique, and gives little indication of the strength of contraction of individual muscles. Many attempts have been made over the years to make it more quantitative, with only limited success. The other problem with EMG is that it may be quite difficult to obtain satisfactory recordings from a walking subject. This depends partly on the electronic characteristics of the equipment being used, and partly on the skill of the operator in selecting the recording sites and in attaching the electrodes to minimize skin resistance and movement artifacts. The EMG signal is generally processed to provide a visible indication of muscle activity.

Despite its limitations, the information provided by EMG on the timing of muscle activation can be of considerable value in gait assessment. For example, one form of treatment in cerebral palsy is to transfer the tendon of a muscle to a different position, thereby altering the action of the muscle. When contemplating this type of surgery, it is essential to use EMG first, to make sure that the timing of muscular contraction is appropriate for its new role.

Energy consumption

The most accurate way of measuring the total amount of energy used in performing an activity such as walking is whole body calorimetry, in which the subject is kept in an insulated chamber, from which the heat output of the body can be measured. This is, of course, quite impractical, except as a research technique. The most usual way of estimating energy expenditure is based on measuring the body's oxygen consumption. There are also less direct methods, using either mechanical calculations or the measurement of heart rate.

Oxygen consumption

The measurement of oxygen consumption requires an analysis of the subject's exhaled breath. If both the volume of exhaled air and its oxygen content are measured, the amount of oxygen consumed in a given time can be calculated. The amount of carbon dioxide produced can also be measured, and the ratio of the carbon dioxide produced to the oxygen consumed (the respiratory quotient) provides information on the type of metabolism that is taking place (aerobic or anaerobic). Except under abnormal environmental conditions it is not necessary to measure either the oxygen or the carbon dioxide in the inspired air, since these are almost constant.

The classic method of measuring oxygen consumption and carbon dioxide production is to fit the subject with a noseclip and mouthpiece, and to collect the whole of the expired air in a large plastic or rubberized canvas Douglas bag or a meteorological balloon. If the subject is walking, some means of following them around with the bag is needed. A small sample of the gas in the bag is then analyzed, after which the volume of exhalate in the bag is measured. After correcting for temperature, air pressure and humidity, a very accurate estimate of oxygen consumption can be obtained. However, collecting the expirate in this way is uncomfortable for the subject, and the technique is quite unsuitable for some patients. A less cumbersome though potentially slightly less accurate method again involves a noseclip and mouthpiece, but uses a portable system which performs continuous gas sampling and volume measurement, so that it is not necessary to collect the whole of the expirate. Either form of gas collection can be achieved using a face mask rather than a mouthpiece and noseclip, although it may be very difficult to prevent leakage or to detect leakage if it does occur. The use of a portable system with a face mask is routine in some gait analysis centers, where analysts find that even children accept it well. Occasionally studies of locomotion are made using a spirometer, in which the subject breathes in and out of an oxygen-filled closed system, which absorbs the exhaled carbon dioxide. Since spirometers are not usually portable, they are practical only when walking on a treadmill.

Mechanical calculations

It was pointed out in Chapter 1 that the expenditure of metabolic energy does not result in the production of an equivalent amount of mechanical work. Indeed, in eccentric muscular activity, metabolic energy is used to absorb, rather than to generate, mechanical energy. Even when muscular contraction is used to do positive work, the efficiency of conversion is relatively low, as well as being variable and difficult to estimate. For these reasons, it is generally unsatisfactory to use mechanical calculations to estimate the total metabolic energy consumed in a complicated activity such as walking. However, this method of estimating energy expenditure is used in some laboratories (Gage *et al.*, 1984), and is known as the 'estimated external work of walking' (EEWW). Calculations of this type are more reliable for activities where the relationship between the muscular contraction and the mechanical output is extremely simple, such as in the concentric contraction of a single muscle.

Even though mechanical calculations are generally unsatisfactory for the estimation of the total energy consumption of the body, the measurement of the energy generation and transfer at individual joints may be of great value in gait analysis. Results of such measurements were given in Chapters 2 and 3. They may be made using combined kinetic/kinematic systems, which are described at the end of this chapter.

Heart rate monitoring

Rose (1983) stated that heart rate monitoring is a good substitute for the measurement of oxygen uptake, since a number of studies over the years have shown that there is a surprisingly close relationship between the two. Heart rate monitoring is certainly much easier to perform, and there are a number of systems available, often based on detecting the pulsatile flow in the capillaries – for example in the finger. Another method of recording heart rate is with the electrocardiogram, using electrodes mounted on the chest. As a general rule, the energy consumption is related to the difference in heart rate between the resting condition and that measured during the exercise. Rather than attempting to relate the change in heart rate directly to energy consumption, some investigators use the physiological cost index (PCI), which is said to be less sensitive to differences between individuals (Steven *et al.*, 1983). It is calculated as follows:

$$PCI = (heart\ rate\ walking - heart\ rate\ resting)/speed$$

The calculation must be made using consistent units, with the heart rate in beats per minute and the speed in meters per minute, or the heart rate in beats per second and the speed in meters per second. The measurement unit for the PCI is net beats per meter. Since the heart rate tends to be somewhat variable, small changes in PCI may not be significant.

Accelerometers

Accelerometers, as their name suggests, measure acceleration. Typically, they contain a small mass connected to a stiff spring, with some electrical means of measuring the spring deflection when the mass is accelerated. The type of accelerometer used in gait analysis is usually very small, weighing only a few grams. It normally only measures acceleration in one direction, but accelerometers may be grouped together for two- or three-dimensional measurements. Solid-state accelerometers, built as integrated circuits, have recently become available. Because of their small size, they may prove to be of value in gait analysis and also in providing feedback for future systems involving powered artificial limbs and orthoses.

Typically, accelerometers have been used for gait analysis in one of two ways – either to measure transient events, or to measure the motion of the limbs.

Measurement of transients

Accelerometers are very suitable for measuring brief, high acceleration events, such as the heelstrike transient. Johnson (1990) described the development of an accelerometer system to assess the performance of shock-attenuating footwear, which has been made available commercially.

The main difficulty with this type of measurement is in obtaining an adequate mechanical linkage between the accelerometer and the skeleton, since slippage occurs in both the skin and the subcutaneous tissues. On a few occasions experiments have been performed with accelerometers mounted on pins and screwed directly into the bones of volunteers. A review of this subject was given by Collins and Whittle (1989).

Measurement of motion

The use of accelerometers for the kinematic analysis of limb motion has been explored by a number of research workers, notably Morris (1973). If the acceleration of a limb segment is known, a single mathematical integration will give its velocity and a second integration its position, providing both position and velocity are known at some point during the measurement period. However, these requirements, combined with the 'drift' from which accelerometers often suffer, has prevented them from coming into widespread use for this purpose. If the limb rotates as well as changes its position, which is usually the case, further accelerometers are needed to measure the angular acceleration.

Gyroscopes

It has been suggested that gyroscopes could be used to measure the orientation of the body segments in space, and that 'rate-gyros' could be used to measure angular velocity and acceleration. Gyroscopes have been used on an experimental basis in some gait laboratories, and the development of very small solid-state devices may make this a useful method of measurement in the future. Nene *et al.* (1999) used a gyroscope, in combination with several accelerometers, in a study of thigh and shank motion during the swing phase of gait.

Figure 4.8 Force platform. Adapted from manufacturer's literature (AMTI Inc).

Force platforms

The force platform, which is also known as a 'forceplate', is used to measure the ground reaction force as a subject walks across it (Fig. 4.8). Although many specialized types of force platform have been developed over the years, most clinical laboratories use a commercial platform, a typical design being about 100 mm high with a flat rectangular upper surface measuring 400 mm by 600 mm. To make the upper surface extremely rigid, it is either made of a large piece of metal or of a light-weight honeycomb structure. Within the platform, a number of transducers are used to measure tiny displacements of the upper surface, in all three axes, when force is applied to it. The electrical output of the platform may be provided as either eight channels or six. An eight-channel output consists of:

1. Four vertical signals, from transducers near the corners of the platform
2. Two fore–aft signals from the sides of the platform
3. Two side-to-side signals, from the front and back of the platform.

A six-channel output generally consists of:

1. Three force vector magnitudes
2. Three moments of force, in a coordinate system based on the center of the platform.

Although it is possible to use the output signal from a force platform directly, for example by displaying it on an oscilloscope, it is much more usual to collect it into a computer through an analog-to-digital converter. Neither the eight-channel nor the six-channel force platform output is particularly convenient for biomechanical calculations, and it is usual to a convert the data to some other form. Regrettably, no standard has been established for the coordinate systems used for either kinetic or kinematic data.

   Ideally a force platform should be mounted below floor level, the upper surface being flush with the floor. If this is not possible, it is usual to build a slightly raised walkway to accommodate the thickness of the platform. It

Figure 4.9 Typical arrangement of two force platforms for use in studies of adults (dimensions in mm).

is highly undesirable to have the subject step up onto the platform and then down off it again, since such a step could never be regarded as 'normal' walking. Force platforms are very sensitive to building vibrations, and many early gait laboratories were built in basements to reduce this form of interference. In the author's opinion this problem has been over-emphasized, since although building vibrations can be seen in force platform data, they are negligible when compared with the magnitude of the signals recorded from subjects walking on the platform.

One problem that may be experienced when using force platforms is that of 'aiming'. To obtain good data, the whole of the subject's foot must land on the platform. It is tempting to tell subjects where the platform is, and to ask them to make sure that their footstep lands squarely on it. However, this is likely to lead to an artificial gait pattern, as the subjects 'aim' for the platform. If at all possible, the platform should be disguised so that it is not noticeably different from the rest of the floor, and subjects should not be informed of its presence. This may require a number of walks to be made, with slight adjustments in the starting position, before acceptable data can be obtained.

Where it is required to record from both feet, the relative positioning of two force platforms can be a considerable problem. There is no single arrangement that is satisfactory for all subjects, and some laboratories have designed systems in which one or both platforms can be moved to suit the gait of individual subjects. Fig. 4.9 shows the arrangement used in a number of laboratories, which is a reasonable compromise for studies on adults, but is unsatisfactory when the stride length is either very short or very long. For subjects who have a very short stride length, such as children, better results may be obtained if the platforms are mounted with their shorter dimensions in the direction of the walk. Alternatively, the direction of the walk may be altered to cross the platforms diagonally. Despite these strategies, the problem may be insoluble. For example, Gage *et al.* (1984) observed that 'force plate data were discounted because the smaller children frequently stepped on the same platform twice because of their short stride lengths'. Some laboratories improve their chances of obtaining good data by using three or four force platforms.

It is often impossible to get the whole of one foot on one force platform and the whole of the other foot on the other one, without also having unwanted additional steps on one or other platform. To some extent computer software can be used to 'unscramble' the data when both feet have stepped on one platform, but more commonly it is necessary to use the data from only one foot at a time.

The usual methods of displaying force platform data are:

1. Individual components, plotted against time (Fig. 2.19)
2. The butterfly diagram (Fig. 2.8)
3. The center of pressure (Figs 2.20 and 2.21).

In the latter case, if it is required to superimpose a foot outline in the correct position on the plot, it is necessary also to measure the position of the foot on the force platform – for example by using talcum powder.

A number of things have to be borne in mind when interpreting force platform data. First, although the foot is the only part of the body in contact with the platform, the forces that are transmitted by the foot are derived from the mass and inertia of the whole body. The force platform has been described as a whole body accelerometer; its output gives the acceleration in three-dimensional space of the center of gravity of the body as a whole, including both the limb that is on the ground and the leg that is swinging through the air. This means that changes in total body inertia may swamp small changes in ground reaction force due to events occurring within the foot. For example, fairly high moments are recorded about the vertical axis during the stance phase of gait (Fig. 4.10). While these may be slightly modified by local events within the foot, they are mainly derived from the acceleration and retardation of the other leg as it goes through the swing phase. The reaction to the forces responsible for this acceleration and retardation are transmitted to the floor through the stance phase leg and appear in the force platform output, principally as a torque about the vertical axis.

When interpreting force platform data, it is also helpful to remember that force is equivalent to the rate of change of momentum. If two objects of identical mass are dropped onto a force platform from the same height, one that bounces will produce a higher ground reaction force than one that does not. This may at first seem surprising, until it is realized that the change in momentum is twice as much for the object that bounces as it is for the one that does not.

It can be difficult to measure transients, such as the heelstrike, using

Figure 4.10 Moments about the vertical axis at the instantaneous center of pressure, during the stance phase of gait. Normal subject, right leg. A positive moment occurs when the foot attempts to move clockwise relative to the floor.

force platforms. This is because the top plate is usually fairly massive, and does not respond well to very brief forces. The heelstrike transient shown in Fig. 2.22 was recorded using a newer design (Bertec) with a stiff but lightweight top plate, giving it a high frequency response. When measuring transients, it is important not to pass the data through a low-pass filter. If the data are sampled using a computer analog-to-digital converter, the sampling rate needs to be high enough to record the waveform accurately (1000 Hz in Fig. 2.22).

Force platform data by themselves are of limited value in gait analysis. Nevertheless, some laboratories use them empirically, for example by looking for particular patterns in the butterfly diagram (Rose, 1985), or comparing the heights of the different peaks and troughs. Some inferences can also be made from the shapes of the curves of the individual force components. For example, there is an association between stance phase flexion of the knee and a dip at mid-stance in the vertical component of force. However, the true value of the force platform is only appreciated when the ground reaction force data are combined with kinematic data. The combination provides a much more complete mechanical description of gait than either by itself, and permits the calculation of joint moments and powers.

A number of workers have developed devices that are not force platforms, but have the same function. Typically, they consist of a small number of force sensors, which are fixed to the sole of a shoe. As the subject walks, the electrical output gives the ground reaction force and the center of pressure. Typically only the vertical component of the ground reaction force is measured, although at least one three-axis system has been described. The advantages claimed are:

1. The ability to measure multiple steps
2. No problems with 'aiming'
3. No risk of stepping on the platform with both feet
4. No risk of missing the platform, either partly or completely.

The disadvantages are the presence of the force sensors beneath the feet, and the associated wiring. The coordinate system for the force measurements moves with the foot, in contrast to the room-based coordinate system used for kinematic data. This makes it very difficult to combine the two types of data, to perform a full biomechanical analysis.

Force platforms may also be used for balance testing and the measurement of postural sway, which are important in some forms of neurological diagnosis. For a complete analysis of the balance mechanism, however, it is necessary to provide some means whereby both the supporting surface and the visual environment may be moved relative to the subject.

Kinematic systems

Kinematics is the measurement of movement, or more specifically the geometric description of motion, in terms of displacements, velocities and accelerations. Kinematic systems are used in gait analysis to record the position and orientation of the body segments, the angles of the joints, and the corresponding linear and angular velocities and accelerations.

Following the pioneering work of Marey and Muybridge in the 1870s, photography remained the method of choice for the measurement of human movement for about 100 years, until it was replaced by electronic systems. Two basic photographic techniques were used – *cine photography* and *multiple-exposure photography*. Cine photography is achieved by the use of a series of separate photographs, taken in quick succession. Multiple exposure photography has existed in many different forms over the years. It is based on the use of a single photograph, or a strip of film, on which a series of images are superimposed, sometimes with a horizontal displacement between each image and the next. The 1960s and 1970s saw the development of gait analysis systems based on *opto-electronic techniques*, including television, and these have now superseded photographic methods.

The general principles of kinematic measurement are common to all systems, and will be discussed before considering particular systems in detail.

General principles

Kinematic measurement may be made in either two dimensions or three. Three-dimensional measurements normally require the use of two or more cameras, although methods have been devised in which a single camera can be used to make limited three-dimensional measurements.

The simplest kinematic measurements are made using a single camera, in an uncalibrated system. Such measurements are fairly inaccurate, but they may be useful for some purposes. Without calibration it is impossible to measure distances accurately, and such a system is normally used only to measure joint angles in the sagittal plane. The camera is positioned at right angles to the plane of motion and as far away as possible, to minimize the distortions introduced by perspective. To give a reasonable size image with a long camera-to-subject distance, a telephoto (long focal length) lens is used. The angles measured from the film are projections of three-dimensional angles onto a two-dimensional plane, and any part of the angulation that occurs out of that plane is ignored. Commercial systems of this type are available for measuring joint angles from television images. Such measurements are subject to yet another form of error, since the horizontal and vertical scales of a television image are often different.

A single-camera system can be used to make approximate measurements of distance if some form of calibration object is used, such as a grid of known dimensions behind the subject. Measurement accuracy will be lost by any movement towards or away from the camera, but this effect can again be minimized if the camera is a long distance away from the subject, using a telephoto lens. Angulations of the limb segments, either towards or away from the camera, will also interfere with length measurements.

To achieve reasonable accuracy in kinematic measurement it is necessary to use a calibrated three-dimensional system, which involves making measurements from more than one viewpoint. Although there are considerable differences in convenience and accuracy between cine film, videotape, television/computer and opto-electronic systems, the data processing for the different types of three-dimensional measurement systems is similar. Almost all commercial kinematic systems use a three-dimensional calibration object, which is viewed by all the cameras. Computer software is used to calculate the relationship between the known three-dimensional positions of markers on the calibration object and the two-dimensional positions of those markers in the fields of view of the different cameras. When a subject walks in front of the cameras, this process is reversed, and three-dimensional positions are calculated for the markers fixed to the subject's limbs, so long as they are visible to at least two cameras. Data are collected at a series of time intervals known as 'frames'. Most systems have an interval between frames of either 20 ms, 16.7 ms or 5 ms, corresponding to data collection frequencies of 50 Hz, 60 Hz or 200 Hz. When a marker can be seen by only one camera, its three-dimensional position cannot be calculated, although it may be estimated by interpolation, using data from earlier and later frames.

All measurement systems, including the kinematic systems to be described, suffer from measurement errors. Measurement accuracy depends to a large extent on the field of view of the cameras, although it also differs somewhat between the different systems. The earlier systems had measurement errors of 2–3 mm in all three dimensions, throughout a volume large enough to cover a complete gait cycle (Whittle, 1982). Recently, design and (especially) calibration improvements have reduced typical errors to less than 1 mm. Some commercial systems claim to provide much higher accuracy than this, but the author treats such claims with skepticism, particularly when applied to the measurement of moving markers under realistic gait laboratory conditions.

Technical descriptions of kinematic systems use, and sometimes misuse, the terms 'resolution', 'precision' and 'accuracy'. In practical terms, *resolution* means the ability of the system to measure small changes in marker position. *Precision* is a measure of system 'noise', being based on the amount of variability there is between one frame of data and the next. For the majority of users, the most important parameter is *accuracy*, which describes the relationship between where the markers really are and where the system says they are!

Most commercial systems are sufficiently accurate to measure the positions of the limbs and the angles of the joints. However, the calculation of linear or angular velocity requires the mathematical differentiation of the position data, which magnifies any measurement errors. A second differentiation is required to determine acceleration, and a small amount of measurement 'noise' in the original data leads to wildly erratic and often unusable results for acceleration. The usual way of avoiding this problem is to smooth the position data, using a low-pass filter, before differentiation. This achieves the desired objective, but means that any genuinely high accelerations, such as that at the heelstrike transient, are lost.

Thus kinematic systems are good at measuring position, but poor at determining acceleration because of the problems of differentiating even slightly noisy data. Conversely, accelerometers are good at measuring acceleration, but poor at estimating position because of the problems of integrating data with baseline drift. Really accurate data could be obtained by combining the two methods, using each to correct the other, and calculating the velocity from both. Some research studies have been conducted using this combined approach.

As well as the errors inherent in measuring the positions of the markers, further errors are introduced because considerable movement may take place between a skin marker and the underlying bone. A few studies have been performed (e.g. Holden *et al.*, 1997; Reinschmidt *et al.*, 1997) in which steel pins have been inserted into the bones of volunteers (usually the investigators themselves) and the positions of skin markers compared with the positions of markers on the pins. The amount of skin movement revealed by such studies is generally somewhat worrying! The amount of error this causes in the final result depends on which parameter is being measured. For example, marker movement has little effect on the sagittal plane knee angle because it causes only a small relative change in the length of fairly long segments, but it may cause considerable errors in transverse plane measurements or in measurements involving shorter segments, such as in the foot. In some cases, the magnitude of the error is greater than the measurement itself! Skin movement may also introduce significant errors in the calculation of joint moments and powers. A possibility for the future is to correct for marker movement by modeling the movement relative to the underlying bone.

A further error is introduced when the positions of the joints are estimated from anthropometric measures (e.g. leg length) and the positions of skin markers, particularly where it is possible to place the markers in the wrong position. Even for subjects with normal anatomy

Figure 4.11 Typical marker configurations for the pelvis and lower limb. Left: using rigid arrays (Cleveland Clinic). Right: skin-mounted, over anatomical landmarks (University of Oxford).

these errors can be substantial; for patients with bony deformity the errors may be even greater. This is a field in which improvements continue to be made.

There are two fundamentally different approaches to positioning markers on the limbs. One method is to mount each marker directly on the skin, generally over a bony anatomical landmark. The position and orientation of the limb segment is then defined by the marker positions. The other approach is to fix a set of at least three markers to each limb segment, either directly or mounted on a rigid structure (sometimes called a pod), so that its position and orientation can be determined in three-dimensional space. The movement of one limb segment relative to the next, and the position of the joint center, may then be derived mathematically. Both methods have advantages and disadvantages, and both suffer from errors due to marker movement. Rigid plates in particular may be moved by the contraction of the underlying muscles, and because they are relatively heavy their inertia causes them to lag behind the limb segment during rapid accelerations. Fig. 4.11 shows two possible ways of arranging lower limb markers, one utilizing pods on the thigh and shank, and one based on markers mounted over anatomical landmarks.

Mention has already been made of the use of force platforms for the measurement of postural sway. Kinematic systems may also be used to make this type of measurement in the standing individual.

Photographic systems

The author does not know of any laboratories that still use multiple-exposure photography, but a few still use cine. The major disadvantages of using cine film are the cost of the materials, the time taken to process the film, and the effort involved in manually digitizing the data. Its advantages are the relatively low cost of the equipment, the potentially high accuracy obtainable, and the ability to film subjects 'in the field' rather than in the laboratory. For this last reason, cine photography is still fairly popular for measuring sporting activities. Normal cine cameras expose at speeds of up to 25 frames per second, but special high-speed cameras are usually needed for gait analysis – and particularly to analyze sporting activities – to avoid blurring of the image and the loss of detail in movements.

The subject is filmed, using one or more cameras, as he or she performs the activity, whether it be walking or performing some sporting event. If a calibration object is being used, this is also filmed, without altering the camera positions or settings. After the film or films have been processed the images are digitized by an operator, who views successive frames, identifies the required landmarks, and measures their two-dimensional co-ordinates. Although this can be done using a ruler, graph paper, or a microscope with a traveling stage, it is most conveniently performed by projecting the film image onto the surface of a 'digitizing tablet' using a specially designed analyzing projector. The operator moves a cursor to the appropriate points in the image, and presses a button to transfer the co-ordinates of each point into a computer. To avoid inaccuracies caused by frame-to-frame variations in film position, it is common also to digitize the positions of fixed markers within the field of view.

Videotape digitizers

The use of videotape to augment visual gait analysis has already been described. Videotape may also be used as the basis for a kinematic system, in the same way that cine photography has been used. It has considerable advantages in terms of cost, convenience and speed, although it may not be quite as accurate because of the poorer resolution of a television image compared with cine film and the further losses involved in recording and replaying videotape. Another considerable advantage, however, is that it is possible to automate the digitization process, using electronic processing of the image, especially if skin markers are used, which show up clearly against the background. A number of commercial systems are available, which can be used either as a two-dimensional system with a single camera or as a three-dimensional system using two or more cameras. Most videotape systems use conventional television equipment, although high-speed systems are also available.

Television/computer systems

A number of different television/computer systems have been developed since 1967. Although the systems differ in detail, the following description is typical.

Figure 4.12 Location of marker centroid (open circle in center) from the position on successive television lines of the leading and trailing edges of the marker image (solid circles).

Reflective markers are fixed to the subject's limbs, either close to the joint centers or to limb segments in such a way as to identify their positions and orientations (Fig. 4.11). Close to the lens of each television camera is an infrared or visible light source, which causes the markers to show up as very bright spots. The markers are usually covered in 'Scotchlite', the material that makes road signs show up brightly when illuminated by car headlights. To avoid the 'smearing' that occurs if the marker is moving, only a short exposure time is used. This may be achieved by one or more of the following:

1. Using stroboscopic illumination
2. Using a mechanical shutter on the camera
3. Using a charge-coupled device (CCD) television camera, which is only enabled (i.e. active) for a short interval during each frame.

If two or more cameras are used, much more accurate measurements can be made if they are synchronized. For normal purposes a conventional television frame rate of 50 Hz or 60 Hz is used, but specialized systems running at higher speeds (typically 200 Hz) are also available. As a general rule, the twin penalties for having the extra speed are increased cost and a reduction in measurement accuracy.

Each television camera is connected to a special interface board that analyzes each television frame. The systems differ in how they locate the centroid, or geometric center, of each marker within the television image, but it is typically calculated using the edges of any bright spots in the field of view (Fig. 4.12). Because a large number of edges are used to calculate the position of the centroid, its position can be determined to a greater accuracy than the horizontal and vertical resolution of the television image. This is known as making measurements with sub-pixel accuracy.

The computer stores the marker centroids from each frame of data for each camera, but initially there is no way to associate a particular marker centroid with a particular physical marker, such as that on the right knee. The process of identifying which marker image is which, for each of the cameras, and of following the markers from one frame of data to the next, is known as tracking or trajectory following. The speed and convenience of this process differs considerably from one system to another, and also between software options from a single manufacturer. In the past this has been the least satisfactory aspect of television/computer systems, although software improvements have now made it much more straightforward. The main differences between systems are in whether the tracking process has to be undertaken separately for each camera, or whether a three-dimensional reconstruction of the data is made before the operator is asked to identify which marker is which. The end result of the tracking and 3-D reconstruction process is a computer file of three-dimensional marker positions.

These systems were originally developed to measure the motion of the lower limbs, but they may also be used to measure motion of the lumbar spine (Whittle and Levine, 1997), the trunk (Crosbie *et al.*, 1997) and the upper limbs. Beyond their use in gait analysis, they are increasingly used to provide the input for computer graphic systems in the video game and motion picture industries.

A number of television/computer systems are also available that were intended for other purposes, such as aircraft tracking, but could possibly be adapted for use in gait analysis. Typically, such systems are based on the identification of particular shapes in the video image.

Active marker systems

Another type of kinematic system uses active markers, typically light-emitting diodes (LEDs), and a special opto-electronic camera. Typically these systems use invisible infra-red radiation, but for the sake of clarity the word 'light' will be used in the following explanation. The camera measures the position of the marker by analyzing the light coming from it. It may be based on either two-dimensional or one-dimensional cameras.

The LEDs are arranged to flash on and off in sequence, so that only one is illuminated at any instant of time. The cameras are thus able to locate each marker in turn, without the need for a tracking procedure to determine which one is which. The penalty for this convenience is the need for the subject to carry a power supply, with wires running to each of the markers. Problems may also occur because the camera records not just the light from the LEDs but also any other light that falls on it. This may include stray ambient light, which is fairly easy to eliminate, but also reflections caused by the markers themselves, which in some systems are difficult both to detect and to eliminate. These problems have led to a decline in the popularity of active marker systems, although they are usually very accurate, have a high sampling rate and are convenient to use.

Other kinematic systems

A number of other methods of making kinematic measurements are in use in different laboratories. Several systems are available which detect the position and orientation of small coils of wire, fixed to a subject's limbs, by means of magnetic fields. For example, Pearcy and Hindle (1989) developed a method for measuring motion of the lumbar spine by mounting a source (transmitter) on the sacrum and a sensor (receiver) over the first lumbar vertebra.

Combined kinetic/kinematic systems

When a kinematic system, such as those described above, is combined with a force platform (which is a kinetic system), the capability of the combined system is greater than that of the sum of its component parts. The reason for this is that if the relationship is known between the limb segments and the ground reaction force vector, it is possible to perform calculations in which the limb is treated as a mechanical system. While not all commercial systems provide the necessary software to make these calculations, there exists the potential to calculate the moments of force and the power generated or absorbed at all the major joints of the lower limb. Such calculations require a knowledge of the masses of the limb segments and the location of their centers of gravity. Direct measurements of these are clearly impossible, but published data, modified to suit the subject's anthropometry, gives an acceptable approximation. It is common practice in such calculations to regard the foot as a single rigid object, although this simplification undoubtedly causes errors in calculating the ankle power.

A fully equipped clinical gait laboratory can be expected to possess, as a minimum, a combined kinetic/kinematic system, with ambulatory EMG (Fig. 4.13), as well as facilities for making videotapes. Equipment may also be available for measuring oxygen uptake or pressure beneath the

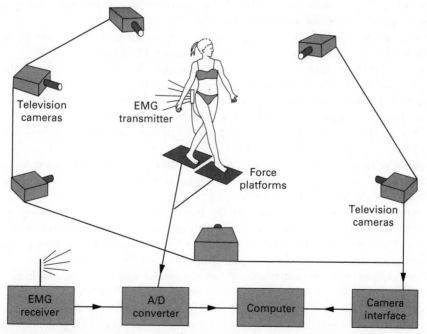

Figure 4.13 The gait analysis equipment used in the author's laboratory, with a six-camera kinematic system, two force platforms and an EMG telemetry system.

feet. If the laboratory is also used for research, then further facilities and equipment may also be present.

One of the big problems with kinetic/kinematic systems is that they provide such a wealth of data that it may be very difficult to distinguish between those observations that are important and those that are not. Recent research has used a number of mathematical, statistical and computational techniques in an attempt to address this problem (Chau, 2001a, 2001b), some examples being multivariate analysis, principal component analysis, neural networks, and the charmingly named 'fuzzy systems'. It may be anticipated that in the future 'expert systems' will be available to draw the attention of clinicians to those aspects of a patient's gait most in need of attention. Another way of coping with this huge quantity of data is to reduce many different measurements to a single index. An example of this is the normalcy index suggested by Schutte *et al.* (2000) as a method of quantifying a patient's disability and providing an outcome measure to gauge the response to treatment.

References and suggestions for further reading

Basmajian JV. (1974) *Muscles Alive: Their Functions Revealed by Electromyography.* Baltimore, MD: Williams & Wilkins.

Brandstater ME, de Bruin H, Gowland C, Clark BM. (1983) Hemiplegic gait: analysis of temporal variables. *Archives of Physical Medicine and Rehabilitation* **64**: 583–587.

Chao EYS. (1980) Justification of triaxial goniometer for the measurement of joint rotation. *Journal of Biomechanics* **13**: 989–1006.

Chau T. (2001a) A review of analytical techniques for gait data. Part 1: fuzzy, statistical and fractal methods. *Gait and Posture* **13**: 49–66.

Chau T. (2001b) A review of analytical techniques for gait data. Part 2: neural network and wavelet methods. *Gait and Posture* **13**: 102–120.

Collins JJ, Whittle MW. (1989) Impulsive forces during walking and their clinical implications. *Clinical Biomechanics* **4**: 179–187.

Crosbie J, Vachalathiti R, Smith R. (1997) Patterns of spinal motion during walking. *Gait and Posture* **5**: 6–12.

Gage JR, Fabian D, Hicks R, Tashman S. (1984) Pre- and postoperative gait analysis in patients with spastic diplegia: a preliminary report. *Journal of Pediatric Orthopedics* **4**: 715–725.

Hillman SJ, Hazlewood ME, Loudon IR, Robb JE. (1998) Can transverse plane rotations be estimated from video tape gait analysis? *Gait and Posture* **8**: 87–90.

Holden JP, Orsini JA, Siegel KL et al. (1997) Surface movement errors in shank kinematics and knee kinetics during gait. *Gait and Posture* **5**: 217–227.

Johnson GR. (1990) Measurement of shock acceleration during walking and running using the shock meter. *Clinical Biomechanics* **5**: 47–50.

Kleissen RFM, Buurke JH, Harlaar J, Zilvold G. (1998) Electromyography in the biomechanical analysis of human movement and its clinical application. *Gait and Posture* **8**: 143–158.

Klenerman L, Dobbs RJ, Weller C et al. (1988) Bringing gait analysis out of the laboratory and into the clinic. *Age and Ageing* **17**: 397–400.

Krebs DE, Edelstein JE, Fishman S. (1985) Reliability of observational kinematic gait analysis. *Physical Therapy* **65**: 1027–1033.

Law HT, Minns RA. (1989) Measurement of the spatial and temporal parameters of gait. *Physiotherapy* **75**: 81–84.

Law HT. (1987) Microcomputer-based, low cost method for measurement of spatial and temporal parameters of gait. *Journal of Biomedical Engineering* **9**: 115–120.

Lord M, Reynolds DP, Hughes JR. (1986) Foot pressure measurement: a review of clinical findings. *Journal of Biomedical Engineering* **8**: 283–294.

Morris JRW. (1973) Accelerometry – a technique for the measurement of human body movements. *Journal of Biomechanics* **6**: 729–736.

Nene A, Mayagoitia R, Veltink P. (1999) Assessment of rectus femoris function during initial swing phase. *Gait and Posture* **9**: 1–9.

New York University (1986) *Lower Limb Orthotics*. New York: Prosthetics and Orthotics, New York University Postgraduate Medical School.

Õunpuu S, DeLuca PA, Bell KJ, Davis RB. (1997) Using surface electrodes for the evaluation of the rectus femoris, vastus medialis and vastus lateralis in children with cerebral palsy. *Gait and Posture* **5**: 211–216.

Pearcy MJ, Hindle RJ. (1989) New methods for the non-invasive three-dimensional measurement of human back movement. *Clinical Biomechanics* **4**: 73–79.

Reinschmidt C, van den Bogert AJ, Lundberg A *et al.* (1997) Tibiofemoral and tibiocalcaneal motion during walking: external vs. skeletal markers. *Gait and Posture* **6**: 98–109.

Robinson JL, Smidt GL. (1981) Quantitative gait evaluation in the clinic. *Physical Therapy* **61**: 351–353.

Rose GK. (1983) Clinical gait assessment: a personal view. *Journal of Medical Engineering and Technology*, **7**: 273–279.

Rose GK. (1985) Use of ORLAU–Pedotti diagrams in clinical gait assessment. *Biomechanical Measurement in Orthopaedic Practice* (M. Whittle, D. Harris, eds), pp. 205–210. Oxford: Clarendon Press.

Saleh M, Murdoch G. (1985) In defence of gait analysis. *Journal of Bone and Joint Surgery* **67B**: 237–241.

Schutte LM, Narayanan U, Stout JL *et al.* (2000) An index for quantifying deviations from normal gait. *Gait and Posture* **11**: 25–31.

Steven MM, Capell HA, Sturrock RD, MacGregor J. (1983) The physiological cost of gait (PCG): a new technique for evaluating nonsteroidal antiinflammatory drugs in rheumatoid arthritis. *British Journal of Rheumatology* **22**: 141–145.

Whittle MW, Levine DF. (1997) Measurement of lumbar lordosis as a component of clinical gait analysis. *Gait and Posture* **5**: 101–107.

Whittle MW. (1982) Calibration and performance of a three-dimensional television system for kinematic analysis. *Journal of Biomechanics* **15**: 185–196.

Zijlstra W, Rutgers AWF, Hof AL, Van Weerden TW. (1995) Voluntary and involuntary adaptation of walking to temporal and spatial constraints. *Gait and Posture* **3**: 13–18.

Technological methods

In the rapidly-changing field of scientific gait analysis, lists of equipment and manufacturers go out of date very quickly. For this reason, readers who need up-to-date information on equipment are encouraged to read recently published journal articles and conference proceedings, and to use the facilities provided by the Internet (see Appendix 3).

5

Applications of gait analysis

The aim of this chapter is to provide a broad overview of some of the ways in which gait analysis is used, particularly in a clinical setting. It is not intended to transform the reader into an expert on the subject. Anyone planning to use gait analysis in clinical decision making should read all of the texts listed at the end of this chapter, attend one or more courses on the interpretation of gait analysis data, and if possible spend some time studying or working in a clinical gait laboratory.

The applications of gait analysis are conveniently divided into two main categories: *clinical gait assessment* and *gait research*. Clinical gait assessment has the aim of helping individual patients directly, whereas gait research aims to improve our understanding of gait, either as an end in itself, or in order to improve medical diagnosis or treatment in the future. There is obviously some overlap, in that many people performing clinical gait assessment use it as the basis for research studies. Indeed, this is the way that most progress in the use of clinical gait assessment is made.

Davis (1988) pointed out that there are considerable differences between the technical requirements for clinical gait assessment and those for gait research. For example, an intrusive measurement system and a cluttered laboratory environment might not worry a fit adult who is acting as an experimental subject, but could cause significant changes in the gait of a child with cerebral palsy. In gait research it might be acceptable to spend a whole day preparing the subject, making the measurements and processing the data, whereas in the clinical setting patients often tire easily and the results are usually needed as quickly as possible. The requirements for accuracy are generally not as great in the clinical setting as they are in the research laboratory, so long as the measurement errors are not large enough to cause a misinterpretation of the clinical condition. However, it is essential that those interpreting the data appreciate the likely magnitude of any such errors. Finally, the system must be able to cope with a wide variety of pathological gaits. It is much easier to make measurements on normal subjects than on those whose gait is very abnormal, which may explain why the literature of the subject is dominated by studies of normal individuals! A final and important point is that there is no value in using a complicated and expensive measurement system unless it provides useful information that cannot be obtained in an easier way.

Gait research may be divided into clinical and fundamental research, the former concentrating on disease processes and methods of treatment and the latter on methods of measurement, and the advancement of knowledge in biomechanics, human performance and physiology. This text will concentrate on clinical gait assessment, and leave further consideration of the subject of gait research for more specialized publications.

Clinical gait assessment

Clinical gait assessment seeks to describe, on a particular occasion, the way in which a person walks. This may be all that is required, if the aim is simply to document a subject's current status. Alternatively, it may be just one step in a continuing process, such as the planning of treatment or the monitoring of progress over a period of time.

Rose (1983) made a distinction between gait analysis and gait assessment. He regarded gait analysis as 'data gathering', and gait assessment as 'the integration of this information with that from other sources for the purposes of clinical decision-making'. This usage of the term 'analysis' differs from that in more technical fields, in which it means 'the processing of data to derive new information'. However, Rose's use of the term is helpful, because it points out that gait assessment is simply one form of clinical assessment. Medical students are taught that clinical assessment is based on three things – history, physical examination and special investigations. In this context gait analysis is simply a special investigation, the results of which will augment other investigations, such as X-ray reports and blood biochemistry, to provide a full clinical picture. The term 'gait evaluation' is sometimes used instead of gait analysis.

The simplest form of gait assessment is practiced every day in orthopedic, physical therapy and rehabilitation clinics throughout the world. Every time doctors or therapists watch a patient walk up and down a room they are performing an assessment of the patient's gait. However, such assessment is often unsystematic, and the most that can be hoped for is to obtain a general impression of how well the patient walks, and perhaps some idea of one or two of the main problems. This could be termed an informal gait assessment. To perform a formal gait assessment requires a careful examination of the gait, using a systematic approach, if possible augmented by objective measurements. Such a gait assessment will usually produce a written report, and the discipline involved in preparing such a report is likely to result in a much more carefully conducted assessment.

The gait analysis techniques that are used in clinical gait assessment vary enormously with the nature of the clinical condition, the skills and facilities available in the individual clinic or laboratory, and the purpose for which the assessment is being conducted. In general, however, clinical gait assessment is performed for one of three possible reasons: it may form the basis of clinical decision making, it may help with the diagnosis of an abnormal gait, or it may be used to document a patient's condition. These will be considered in turn.

Clinical decision making

Both Rose (1983) and Gage (1983) suggested that clinical decision making in cases of gait abnormality should involve three clear stages:

1. *Gait assessment*: this starts with a full clinical history, both from the patient and from any others involved, such as doctors, therapists or family members. Where a patient has previously had surgery, details of this should be obtained, if possible from the operative notes. History taking is followed by a physical examination, with particular emphasis on the musculoskeletal system. In many laboratories, physical examinations are performed by both a doctor and a physical therapist. Finally, a formal gait analysis is carried out.

2. *Hypothesis formation*: the next stage is the development of a hypothesis regarding the cause or causes of the observed abnormalities. Time needs to be set aside to review the data, and consultation between colleagues, particularly those from different disciplines, is extremely valuable. Indeed, almost all of those using gait assessment as a clinical decision-making tool stress the value of this team approach. In forming a hypothesis as to the fundamental problem in a patient with a gait disorder, Rose (1983) emphasized that the patient's gait pattern is not entirely the direct result of the pathology, but is the net result of the original problem and the patient's ability to compensate for it. He observed that the worse the underlying problem the easier it is to form a hypothesis, since the patient is less able to compensate.

3. *Hypothesis testing*: this stage is sometimes omitted, when there is little doubt as to the cause of the abnormalities observed. However, where some doubt does exist the hypothesis can be tested in two different ways – either by using a different method of measurement, or by attempting in some way to modify the gait. Some laboratories routinely use a fairly complete standard protocol, including videotape, kinematic measurement, force platform measurements and surface EMG. They will then add other measurements, such as fine-wire EMG, where this is necessary to test a hypothesis. Other clinicians start the gait analysis using a simple method, such as videotape, and only add other techniques, such as EMG or the use of a force platform, where they would clearly be helpful. Rose (1983) opposed the use of a standard protocol for all patients, since some of the procedures turn out to have been unnecessary and there is a risk of ending up with 'an exhausted subject in pain'. The other method of testing a hypothesis is to re-examine the gait after attempting some form of modification, typically by the application of an orthosis to limit joint motion, or by paralyzing a muscle using local anaesthetic. The ultimate form of gait modification is the surgical operation, with retesting following recovery. However, this is a rather drastic form of hypothesis testing, which can be used only where there is a good reason to suppose that the operation will lead to a definite improvement.

Different types of gait analysis data may be useful for different aspects of the gait assessment. Information on foot timing may be useful to identify asymmetries, and may indicate problems with balance and stability. The general gait parameters give a guide to the degree of disability, and may be used to monitor progress or deterioration with the passage of time. The kinematics of limb motion describe abnormal movements, but do not identify the 'guilty' muscles.

The most useful measures are probably the joint moments and joint powers, particularly if this information is supplemented by EMG data. Hemiparetic patients may show greater differences between the two sides in muscle power output than in any of the other measurable parameters, including EMG. Winter (1985) stressed the need to work backwards from the observed gait abnormalities to the underlying causes in terms of the 'guilty' motor patterns, using both the EMG and the moments about the hip, knee and ankle joints. He offered a method of charting gait abnormalities, and a table giving the common gait disorders, their possible causes, and the type of evidence that would confirm or refute them (Table 5.1). Although the next step, that of treatment, was not considered in detail, he suggested that once an accurate diagnosis had been made, the therapist would be challenged to 'alter or optimize the abnormal motor patterns'.

Many others working in the field of clinical gait assessment have noted the difficulty of deducing the underlying cause from the observed gait abnormalities, because of the compensations that take place. A number of attempts have been made to simplify this process by using a systematic approach. Computer-based expert systems are very suitable for this type of application, and a number of such systems have already been developed for clinical gait assessment. Since gait patterns are seldom clear cut, such expert systems cannot generally use a fixed set of rules, but rather need to learn to recognize patterns within complex sets of data. Techniques such as neural networks and fuzzy logic are being explored for this purpose (Chau, 2001). No doubt the number and quality of such systems will increase in the future.

The following paragraphs describe how gait assessment is used for clinical decision making in a typical laboratory. The details will, of course, differ from one laboratory to another, based on the skills and interests of the laboratory personnel, the facilities and equipment available, and the types of patient seen.

When the patient arrives at the facility a thorough history is obtained, and a physical examination is performed by both a physician and a physical therapist. Height, weight, and a number of other measurements are made. The patient's gait is recorded on videotape, viewing the patient from both sides, and from the front and back. The technological element of the gait analysis is performed, using a television/computer kinematic system, and one or more force platforms. The number of cameras used is dictated largely by economics. Ideally at least six cameras should be used, but three can give acceptable data, particularly if measurements are made from only one side of the body at a time. Most laboratories record surface EMG, either on muscles which are selected on a case-by-case basis, or on a standard set, such as the anterior gluteals, gluteus maximus, quadriceps, medial and lateral hamstrings, triceps surae, tibialis anterior and the hip adductors. Depending on the clinical condition, fine-wire EMG of selected muscles may be recorded, either at the same time or later. For example, Gage *et al.* (1984) reported that where a hip flexion contracture is present,

Table 5.1 Common gait abnormalities, their possible causes, and evidence required for confirmation (reproduced, with permission, from Winter, 1985)

Foot slap at heel contact	Below normal dorsiflexor activity at heel contact	Below normal tibialis anterior EMG or dorsiflexor moment at heel contact
Forefoot or flatfoot initial contact	(a) Hyperactive plantarflexor activity in late swing (b) Structural limitation in ankle range (c) Short step-length	(a) Above normal plantarflexor EMG in late swing (b) Decreased dorsiflexor range of motion (c) See (a), (b), (c) and (d) immediately below
Short step	(a) Weak push off prior to swing (b) Weak hip flexors at toe off and early swing (c) Excessive deceleration of leg in late swing (d) Above normal contralateral hip extensor activity during contralateral stance	(a) Below normal plantarflexor moment or power generation (A2) or EMG during push off (b) Below normal hip flexor moment or power or EMG during late push off and early swing (c) Above normal hamstring EMG or knee flexor moment or power absorption (K4) late in swing (d) Hyperactivity in EMG of contralateral hip extensors
Stiff-legged weight-bearing	Above normal extensor activity at the ankle, knee or hip early in stance*	Above normal EMG activity or moments in hip extensors, knee extensors or plantarflexors early in stance
Stance phase with flexed but rigid knee	Above normal extensor activity in early and mid-stance at the ankle and hip, but with reduced knee extensor activity	Above normal EMG activity or moments in hip extensors, and plantarflexors in early and mid-stance
Weak push off accompanied by observable pull off	Weak plantarflexor activity at push off. Normal, or above normal, hip flexor activity during late push off and early swing or moment or power during late push off and early swing	Below normal plantarflexor EMG, moment or power (A2) during push off. Normal or above normal hip flexor EMG
Hip hiking in swing (with or without circumduction of lower limb)	(a) Weak hip, knee or ankle dorsiflexor activity during swing (b) Overactive extensor synergy during swing	(a) Below normal tibialis anterior EMG or hip or knee flexors during swing (b) Above normal hip or knee extensor EMG or moment during swing
Trendelenburg gait	(a) Weak hip abductors (b) Overactive hip adductors	(a) Below normal EMG in hip abductors: gluteus medius and minimus, tensor fascia lata (b) Above normal EMG in hip adductors, adductor longus, magnus and brevis, and gracilis

* Note: there may be below normal extensor forces at one joint but only in the presence of abnormally high extensor forces at one or both of the other joints.

his laboratory routinely records fine-wire EMG from the iliopsoas. Some facilities record kinetic, kinematic and EMG data at the same time; others find it more convenient to record EMG separately.

Since great variability may exist between one walk and another, any single walk may not be representative, particularly if patients hesitate or momentarily lose their balance. For this reason, a number of walks are recorded and the results examined for consistency. Depending on the clinical status of the patient, walks may be made under a number of different conditions, for example with and without shoes, with or without an orthosis, or using different walking aids.

Once preliminary reports on the history and physical examination have been prepared, the data processed and charts printed, the team meets to discuss the case. The composition of the team varies considerably from one facility to another, but it would commonly consist of a physician, a physical therapist and a kinesiologist or bioengineer, with the optional addition of other physicians, physical therapists, prosthetists and ortho-tists. Indeed, anyone with an interest in providing the best possible care for the patient may be invited to join the team to discuss a particular patient. In many facilities the team includes the orthopaedic surgeon who will ultimately perform any necessary surgery.

The assessment begins with a careful review of the patient's history, and the examinations by the physician and physical therapist. The gait videotapes are watched and discussed, and notes are made for inclusion in a final report. The general gait parameters are noted, to determine the degree of disability and the effects of any changes in conditions, such as orthoses or walking aids. Different gait analysis systems provide different amounts of technical data on the patient's gait, and examination of the charts can be a long and painstaking process. One of the most important parts of the assessment is to identify deviations from normal in the joint angles, and to determine the cause of such deviations. This process is easier if joint moments and powers are available. Joint moments indicate in general terms which structures in the region of a joint are coming under tension, and the degree of tension in them. Joint powers may help to discriminate between concentric muscle contraction, eccentric muscle contraction and passive tension in soft tissues. They can also distinguish between powerful and weak muscle contractions. The EMG also contributes to this process by identifying which muscles are electri-cally active, and are thus candidates for developing tension, at different times during the gait cycle.

Very briefly, interpretation of the gait analysis charts may involve the following steps:

1. *Joint angle*: what is the angle of a joint at a particular part of the gait cycle, and in which direction is it moving?
2. *Joint moment*: is the internal moment extensor or flexor? This will indicate what muscles or ligaments are under tension, and to what degree.
3. *Joint power*: is power generation or absorption taking place? This would indicate concentric or eccentric contraction, or storage and release of energy by stretching elastic tissues.

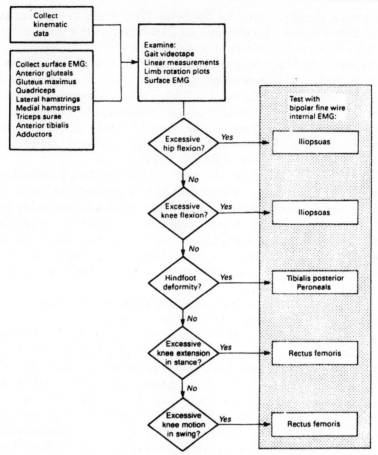

Figure 5.1 Gait assessment flowchart, used for selecting muscles for testing with fine-wire EMG (Davis, 1988).

4. *EMG*: is the muscle electrical activity consistent with the kinematic data?

At this time, a hypothesis is formed as to the detailed cause of any gait abnormalities present. This may indicate a need for further data, such as fine-wire EMG recordings from other muscles (Fig. 5.1), and the patient may be asked to return for further tests. Having made a detailed diagnosis of the patient's functional problems, an appropriate form of treatment is decided, which in many cases involves surgery. In such cases, the final stage of assessment would be an examination under anesthetic made just prior to the commencement of surgery. The muscle relaxant used with the anesthetic abolishes spasticity, and makes it possible to distinguish between structural abnormalities, such as contractures, and the effects of muscle tension. If the treatment selected involves physical therapy or the use of an orthosis, the patient would be monitored during the course of such treatment to determine whether the initial decisions were appropriate.

Once treatment has been carried out, and after a suitable recovery period, a further gait assessment is often performed. The purpose of this is first to determine the success of the treatment, and secondly to decide whether the patient would benefit from further surgery, physical therapy or orthotic prescription. It also gives the clinical team the opportunity to perform a critical review of the original diagnosis and treatment plan, to decide whether the correct decisions were made. If an error has been made it is important to recognize it and to learn from it, to prevent it from happening again. There is usually no change in EMG postoperatively, and the main criteria for determining the success (or otherwise) of treatment are the general gait parameters and the joint rotations. In subjects in whom it can be measured from the kinematic data, the estimated external work of walking (EEWW) may also be used as a measure of improvement. According to Gage, total body energy consumption is the best measure of the success of treatment. Perry uses three criteria to gauge success: walking speed, energy consumption and cosmesis.

Diagnosis of abnormal gait

Most patients undergoing gait assessment have already been diagnosed, as far as the principal disease or condition affecting them is concerned. In such cases, gait assessment is carried out to make a more detailed diagnosis, relating to the exact state of particular joints and muscles. On occasion, however, a patient is seen in whom the cause of an abnormal gait is not clear.

A number of apparently abnormal gait patterns are, in fact, habits rather than the result of underlying pathology, and the techniques of gait analysis may be useful to identify them. Since any pathology affecting the locomotor system generally reduces a person's ability to alter his or her gait pattern, a variable gait may be suggestive of a habit pattern, and a highly reproducible gait may suggest a pathological process. However, the assessment must take many other factors into account, including the possibility of a pathological process that includes an element of variability, such as ataxia or athetosis.

An example of the use of gait assessment to differentiate between pathological gaits and habit patterns is in the diagnosis of toe walking. Some children prefer to walk on their toes rather than on the whole foot, in a pattern known as idiopathic toe walking. It is important, but also quite difficult, to differentiate between this relatively harmless and self-limiting condition and more serious conditions, such as cerebral palsy. Hicks *et al.* (1988) stated that earlier attempts to establish the diagnosis, using EMG alone, had not been successful. In their study, they compared the gait kinematics of seven idiopathic toe-walkers and seven children with mild spastic diplegia. There was a clear difference between the two groups in the pattern of sagittal plane knee and ankle motion. Both groups had initial contact either by the flat foot or by toestrike, but in the case of the toe walkers this was due to ankle plantarflexion, whereas in the children with cerebral palsy it was due to knee flexion. There were also other differences between the two groups, suggesting that gait assessment would be very helpful in making a differential diagnosis.

Documentation of a patient's condition

Although clinical decision making is the most direct way in which gait assessment may be used to help an individual patient, there are also instances when simply documenting the current state of a patient's gait may be of value. For some purposes, such documentation may be needed only on a single occasion, where the aim is to quantify a patient's disability. For other purposes, a series of gait assessments over a period of time may be used to monitor either progress or deterioration.

As part of the overall assessment of a patient with a disability, a clinician may require more detail about how well the patient walks. This type of gait assessment may be directly intended for use in clinical decision making, but it is sometimes performed speculatively, in case it should reveal a treatable cause for the patient's walking disorder.

Gait assessment is frequently used to document the progress of a patient undergoing some form of treatment. The results of the assessment may be used to identify areas where the treatment is ineffective, or it may define an end point for stopping treatment, when progress appears to have ceased. Another use of this type of serial assessment is to convince the patient and relatives that progress has been made, when their own faulty recollection tells them it has not. An objective form of monitoring progress is particularly important for use in the evaluation of novel and controversial methods of treatment, where the enthusiasm of the investigators has been known to lead to errors of judgement!

Gait assessment may form part of the overall documentation of a number of medical conditions that involve the locomotor system. A deterioration in gait with the passage of time may be detected early, allowing remedial action to be taken. It may also identify clinical signs that should be looked for in other cases of the same condition, particularly if it is very uncommon.

The shape of ground reaction force curve is sometimes used empirically to monitor progress in rehabilitation. It has been observed that patients walking slowly and painfully have a flat-topped curve, which gradually changes towards the double-peaked normal curve (Fig. 2.19) as their condition improves.

A regrettable but inescapable part of medical practice today is concerned with litigation. The ability of gait assessment to measure objectively at least some aspects of disability makes it very useful in supporting claims for damages. The author was the first person to present gait analysis data as evidence in a court of law in the United Kingdom, in a case in which a child suffered spastic hemiplegia as a result of a motor vehicle accident. Another aspect of litigation concerns medical practice itself, and the risk that a doctor or other health care professional may be sued for negligence. Now that gait assessment has shown its value in the management of cerebral palsy, it may only be a matter of time before it is considered unwise to operate on a patient with cerebral palsy without a preoperative gait assessment.

Conditions benefiting from gait assessment

A large number of diseases affect the neuromuscular and musculoskeletal systems, and may thus lead to disorders of gait. Among the most important are:

1. Cerebral palsy
2. Parkinsonism
3. Muscular dystrophy
4. Osteoarthritis
5. Rheumatoid arthritis
6. Lower limb amputation
7. Stroke
8. Head injury
9. Spinal cord injury
10. Myelodysplasia
11. Multiple sclerosis.

While it is possible that gait assessment may benefit a person affected by any one of these conditions, it is clear that greater benefits are possible in some pathologies than in others. This chapter will end with a consideration of those conditions for which there is good evidence that gait assessment is worthwhile.

Cerebral palsy

According to Rose (1983), decision making in cerebral palsy may be 'significantly affected' by the results of gait assessment, making this condition one of the most important practical applications of the methodology. A very good case for this was made by Gage (1983), who studied the variable outcome normally seen following the surgical treatment of spastic diplegia, and ascribed it to the fact that 'the spectrum of neurological pathology cannot be differentiated by clinical evaluation alone'.

It is probable that, in the whole world, no more than a few thousand sufferers from cerebral palsy have received any systematic form of gait assessment prior to surgical treatment. However, the medical community is gradually coming to accept that better treatment decisions can be made with the benefit of gait assessment, and new gait labs are being opened all the time.

Gage (1983) also pointed out the desirability of performing all the necessary surgical corrections in a single operative session. Although there are considerable benefits to the patient from having all their operations at once, there is also a risk that it will 'increase the likelihood of a judgement error' (Gage *et al.*, 1984). For this reason, this approach can only be used safely if accurate and complete diagnostic information is available, based on a very thorough gait assessment. Most centers prefer to delay assessment until the gait has matured, generally between the ages of 6 and 8 years (Gage *et al.*, 1984).

It is essential in cerebral palsy to distinguish between the primary pathology and the patient's coping responses. A significant proportion of children undergoing surgery for cerebral palsy are made worse rather than better, because inappropriate treatment removes their ability to compensate. For example, a child may be vaulting on one side because of an inability to flex the opposite knee in the swing phase. If the vaulting is erroneously ascribed to a tight heel cord, and treated by a heel cord lengthening, the gait would be made worse, not better. Regrettably, errors of this type are all too common, particularly when treatment is prescribed without the benefit of gait assessment.

Of particular importance in the management of cerebral palsy is a knowledge of the activity of particular muscles, both to pinpoint 'guilty' muscles and to decide whether a muscle is suitable for transplantation. Chong *et al.* (1978) studied the problem of internal rotation of the leg while walking, in children with cerebral palsy. They demonstrated the value of ambulatory EMG measurements in determining whether or not there was phasic overactivity of the medial hamstrings. As always in cerebral palsy, a number of different patterns of muscle activity were found in subjects who appeared to be similar in other respects. They observed that some patients had tightness of the medial hamstrings when walking but not on clinical examination, and considered that this cause of an internal rotation gait would be 'almost impossible to detect without electromyography'. They found other patients who had tight hamstrings on clinical examination, but in whom there was no EMG evidence of phasic overactivity. In these patients, they stated that hamstring lengthening would not correct the gait abnormality and that, if the internal rotation was severe enough, a derotation osteotomy of the femur was indicated. In current practice, the main indication for hamstring lengthening is persistent knee flexion in the stance phase of gait.

Baumann and Hanggi (1977) showed that gait assessment, using EMG, could distinguish between muscle paralysis and incorrect phasing of muscle contraction. This becomes important when considering transplanting a muscle tendon to another site to replace a muscle action which is deficient. This can be a very useful method of treatment in cerebral palsy, but it is vital to know the phasic activity of a muscle before transplanting it. As a general rule, the phasic activity of muscles in cerebral palsy is fixed, with no possibility of re-education, so that if muscle activity is required during the stance phase, the surgery will be doomed to failure if the transposed muscle is only active during swing.

Gage *et al.* (1987) reported good results from an operation to correct the stiff-legged gait seen in some children with cerebral palsy. Dynamic EMG is essential to identify those who would benefit from the procedure, which is appropriate only for those in whom there is contraction of the quadriceps throughout the swing phase. The operation, which was suggested by Perry (1987), involves transfer of the rectus femoris to behind the knee on either the medial or the lateral side (Chung et al., 1997), in connection with lengthening of the hamstrings. This operation is commonly performed when the peak of knee flexion in the swing phase is both delayed and reduced in magnitude, and where there is EMG evidence of rectus femoris activity during swing.

Winters *et al.* (1987) described their use of clinical gait assessment to decide the optimal treatment for patients with spastic diplegia, which may result from cerebral palsy or a number of other conditions. Their use of gait assessment to classify spastic diplegia into four clinical groups, each of which benefits from a different type of treatment, was described in Chapter 3.

An examination of the moments of force about the joints may explain some of the gait abnormalities in cerebral palsy, since deformity may reduce the muscle lever arms, requiring very high muscle forces to be produced in order to produce modest joint moments.

The following kinematic abnormalities are commonly seen in cerebral palsy (Walsh *et al.*, 1993):

1. Internal rotation of the hip
2. Limited extension of the hip in stance
3. Excessive anterior pelvic tilt
4. A biphasic pattern of pelvic sagittal plane motion due to hip flexor spasticity – the so-called 'double-bump' pattern of pelvic motion.

A number of studies have described kinetic abnormalities in cerebral palsy (Gage, 1994; Õunpuu *et al.*, 1996; Lin *et al.*, 2000). Typical abnormalities are as follows:

1. The internal hip moment changes from extensor to flexor later than normal when there is overactivity of the hip flexor muscles
2. Equinus foot deformity produces knee extension or hyperextension, through a plantarflexion/knee extension couple
3. Persistent internal knee extension moment, due to excessive knee flexion (crouch gait)
4. Reduced ankle plantarflexor power generation
5. The internal ankle moment may show a biphasic plantarflexor moment, due to clonus of the gastrocnemius – the so-called 'double-bump' pattern of ankle moment.

Both Gage (1991) and Perry (1992) have given excellent examples of the ways in which gait assessment may help in the management of individuals with cerebral palsy, and progress continues to be made in this regard, especially through the interpretation of joint moments and powers. Since the neurological deficit is permanent and irreparable, the timing of muscular contraction cannot be altered by treatment. However, the gait of a person with cerebral palsy can often be improved considerably in other ways, the main forms of treatment being:

1. Using dorsal rhizotomy to reduce muscle tone, by destroying a proportion of the sensory fibers as they enter the spinal cord
2. Changing the mode of action of a muscle by tendon transplantation, e.g. changing rectus femoris into a knee flexor
3. Correcting bony misalignments, e.g. tibial or femoral rotational osteotomy
4. Strengthening a muscle by training
5. Making a muscle weaker or non-functional by lengthening or cutting its tendon, e.g. Achilles tendon lengthening
6. Lengthening a muscle by stretching, using serial casting and/or night splints

7. Lengthening a muscle by stretching, after paralyzing it by an injection of botulinum toxin (the effects of which last for several months), often combined with serial casting (Graham *et al.*, 2000)
8. Using an orthosis to limit the movement of a joint, or to apply a force in a particular direction, e.g. ankle–foot orthosis (AFO) to control foot drop
9. Using drug treatment to reduce spasticity, e.g. oral baclofen
10. Using an implanted pump to infuse drugs into the space around the spinal cord, to reduce spasticity, e.g. intrathecal baclofen.

The management of individuals with cerebral palsy, with the aid of gait analysis, has developed considerably since about 1980, and it has an extensive literature of its own, which should be consulted for further information. The references cited above should provide a suitable entry point into this literature.

Gait disorders of the elderly

Cunha (1988) discussed the gait of the elderly, and pointed out that many pathological gait disorders are incorrectly thought to be part of the normal aging process. Identification of an underlying cause, which may be treatable, could result in an improved life for the patient, and a reduced risk of falls and fractures. Cunha classified the causes of the gait disorders of old age as follows: neurological, psychological, orthopedic, endocrinological, general, drugs, senile gait and associated conditions. He described the features of the gait in many conditions affecting the elderly, and suggested a plan for the investigation and management of these patients.

Other conditions

A number of other possible uses for gait assessment in clinical decision making have been suggested over the years. In most cases, the publications dealing with these applications have been largely descriptive, with examples of clinical applications, such as the following.

Rose (1983) suggested that gait analysis was useful in the assessment of patients with multiple joint disease. He cited the case of a woman with a stiff but painless hip on one side, and a painful deformed knee on the other. Gait analysis showed that the stiff hip was causing abnormal loading in the painful knee, suggesting that total knee joint replacement would be 'doomed to early failure'. The recommended course of action was to perform an operation to improve the mobility of the hip before attempting any surgery on the knee. Rose did not, however, see any great value in performing gait assessment on patients requiring the replacement of only a single joint.

Prodromos *et al.* (1985) investigated the variable clinical results that follow the operation of high tibial osteotomy for osteoarthritis of the knee with a varus deformity. They found that clinical success or failure could be predicted by the preoperative measurement of the frontal plane moment of force at the knee, those patients with a high moment having a significantly worse result, with a recurrence of deformity, than those with a low moment.

Patients with a rupture of the anterior cruciate ligament in the knee may show altered muscle activity, for example an increase in the activity of the hamstrings. EMG of these muscles could be used either as a diagnostic aid or to monitor the results of ligament replacement surgery. Berchuck *et al.* (1990) reported a 'quadriceps avoidance' pattern, in which individuals with a ruptured anterior cruciate ligament lacked the normal internal knee extension moment provided by quadriceps contraction. Roberts *et al.* (1999) later challenged this finding, which may relate more to knee pain than to the absence of the anterior cruciate ligament.

The management of hemiplegia may be enhanced if a careful assessment of a patient's gait is performed. This may be used as a basis for planning either physical therapy (New York University, 1986) or some form of surgical treatment. Hemiplegic patients tend to walk very inefficiently, so that measuring their joint moments and powers may suggest ways in which training could be used to reduce their energy expenditure. Waters *et al.* (1979) used fine-wire electrodes to measure the EMG activity of all four heads of the quadriceps muscle, in hemiplegic patients with a stiff-legged gait. If there was overactivity in only one or two components of the muscle, during late stance phase and early swing, good results were obtained by performing appropriate tenotomies.

Other neurological conditions could also benefit from the information provided by gait assessment. For example, Rose (1983) stated that gait assessment can make a significant contribution to the management of muscular dystrophy.

Lord *et al.* (1986) suggested that the measurement of pressure beneath the foot could play a useful part in patient management by making it possible to provide custom-made pressure-relieving insoles. The manufacture of these insoles could be achieved either by a craftsman, using information provided by the measurement system, or automatically by some form of computer-aided design and manufacture (CAD-CAM). Having produced the insoles, further pressure measurements could then be used to check their effectiveness. Force platforms have also been used as an aid in the prescription of corrective footwear, by measuring the symmetry of the force patterns between the two feet. Pressure distribution beneath the foot could also be used to monitor the results of treatment for various types of foot disorder, such as a fracture involving the subtalar joint.

A high proportion of longstanding diabetics develop peripheral neuropathy, and many of these go on to develop pressure sores on the feet. Regrettably, these may not be detected until deep-seated infection has occurred, which often leads to amputation, and occasionally to death. The detection of these pressure sores does not need gait assessment – it merely needs someone to inspect the feet on a regular basis. However, the detection of high pressures, before ulceration has occurred, can be achieved by a pressure measurement system. Cavanagh *et al.* (1985) described a method that could be used to detect areas of dangerously high pressure beneath the feet of diabetic patients, prior to the actual formation of an ulcer. Other groups of patients who might benefit from foot pressure mon-

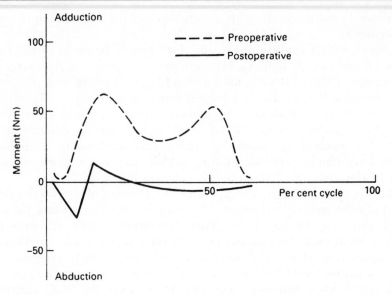

Figure 5.2 Change in frontal plane external knee moment from excessive adduction
moment to abnormally low biphasic moment, following high tibial osteotomy (Jefferson and Whittle, 1989).

itoring are those with peripheral neuropathy from other causes, such as
Hansen's disease (leprosy), and people with severely deformed feet, for
example from rheumatoid arthritis.

In many other conditions affecting gait, the use of gait analysis techniques, particularly the more advanced methods involving the measurement
of moments and powers, gives a better insight into the exact nature of the
deficit and the way in which the patient is able to compensate for it. This
may lead to a better understanding of the pathological condition itself, and
may also suggest improved methods of treatment. For example, if a patient
is compensating for weakness of one muscle group by using other muscles,
physical therapy could be aimed at strengthening those muscles, and
perhaps at increasing the patient's skill in using these slightly unnatural
movements.

As well as its use in comparative trials between two or more forms of
treatment, gait analysis is also commonly used simply to quantify the
benefit that a patient receives from a particular type of treatment. In
such cases, a comparison may be made with pre-treatment data values
for that patient, and with comparable results from normal individuals.
Fig. 5.2 shows an example of how the operation of high tibial osteotomy
was successful in eliminating an excessively high external adduction
moment at the knee (Jefferson and Whittle, 1989).

Gait assessment may be of value in the disciplines of prosthetics and
orthotics. The alignment and adjustment of prosthetic limbs may be
improved using objective measurements of gait, particularly if repeat
trials are performed with different adjustments. Orthotic prescription
may be improved if the gait is monitored with the patient wearing
different types or configurations of orthosis, for example with different
ankle alignments on an ankle–foot orthosis for drop foot (Lehmann *et al.*,

1987). Trials of different orthoses may also form part of the process of hypothesis testing described above (Õunpuu *et al.*, 1996).

The design and prescription of orthoses tends to be based much more on art than science, and a significant proportion of orthotic devices are regrettably not used by the patients for whom they are made. Gait analysis is able to provide an insight into the functioning of orthoses, and to compare different designs. It may also permit improvements to be made to existing designs, such as the Saltiel anterior floor reaction orthosis (Harrington *et al.*, 1984). Some objective studies of orthoses have failed to demonstrate that they have any significant mechanical effects. It then becomes arguable whether the devices really do have no effect, or whether their mode of action is too subtle for the methods of measurement being used.

Gait analysis can be used for the assessment of new or modified forms of lower limb prosthesis. It may be used to examine the effects of changing the design of a prosthetic limb, such as by altering the mass distribution (Tashman *et al.*, 1985), or using knee joints with different types of braking mechanism (Hicks *et al.*, 1985). Two types of measurement are of particular value in this type of assessment – the kinematics of motion and the muscle moments and powers the amputee has to produce in order to walk.

Measurement of the power output across the ankle joint is very valuable when comparing different prosthetic foot mechanisms. One of the major differences between the prosthetic foot and the natural foot is the inability of the prosthetic foot to generate power during pre-swing (third rocker). However, it is able to store energy during the second rocker and to release it during the third rocker, which may lead to a more natural gait pattern. Gait analysis can be used to examine the energy storage and recovery by prosthetic foot mechanisms, and to determine how well particular types of foot suit different categories of patient. For example, a young subject who has suffered a traumatic amputation is much better able to take advantage of an energy-storing foot mechanism than an elderly subject who has received an amputation for vascular disease.

Future developments

Gait analysis has advanced significantly since joint moments and powers have become routinely available. What would be of even more value, if it could be provided, would be knowledge of the forces in the different structures in and around the joints. The use of mathematical modeling permits estimates to be made of forces in the tendons and ligaments, and across the articular surfaces. Unfortunately, a large number of unknown factors are involved, particularly the internal moment generated by the different muscles and the extent of any co-contraction by antagonistic muscles. For this reason such calculations can only be approximate, but they may nonetheless be extremely valuable, particularly in clinical and biomechanical research. The output of mathematical models may be further refined using EMG. Most models offer a range of possible solutions, based on different combinations of active muscles. Even though it is not generally possible to convert EMG signals directly into muscle contraction force, the

knowledge that a muscle is either inactive, contracting a little or contracting strongly, may make it possible to eliminate at least some of the possible
model solutions, and thereby to improve the reliability of the results.

Conclusion

Gait analysis has had a long history, and for much of this time it has
remained an academic discipline with little practical application. This
situation has now changed, and the value of the methodology has been
unequivocally demonstrated in certain conditions, particularly cerebral
palsy. We are already seeing a decrease in the cost and complexity of
kinematic systems, and an increasing acceptance by clinicians of the
results of gait analysis. This trend will hopefully continue so that the
use of these techniques will increase, both in those conditions for which
its value is already recognized and in a variety of other conditions.

Although the current text has focused on gait analysis, this type of
measurement equipment may also be used for other purposes – a fact
that may be relevant to those trying to obtain funds to set up a gait
analysis laboratory! The use of force platforms and kinematic systems
for balance and posture testing has been referred to, as has their use in
studying performance in a wide range of sports. Clinical studies have also
been made of people standing up, sitting down, starting and stopping
walking, ascending and descending stairs. The equipment has been used
to measure the movements of the back, not only in walking but also in the
standing and sitting positions. It has also been used to monitor the
movements of the upper limbs, both in athetoid patients and in
ergonomic studies of reach. Walking is only one of many things that can
be done by the musculoskeletal system. It is only sensible to broaden our
horizons, and to use the power of the modern measurement systems to
study a wide range of other activities.

References and suggestions for further reading

Baumann JU, Hanggi A. (1977) A method of gait analysis for daily orthopaedic
practice. *Journal of Medical Engineering and Technology* **1**: 86–91.

Berchuck M, Andriacchi TP, Bach BR, Reider B. (1990) Gait adaptations by
patients who have a deficient anterior cruciate ligament. *Journal of Bone and
Joint Surgery* **72A**: 871–877.

Cavanagh PR, Hennig EM, Rodgers MM, Sanderson DJ. (1985) The measurement of
pressure distribution on the plantar surface of diabetic feet. *Biomechanical
Measurement in Orthopaedic Practice* (M. Whittle, D. Harris, eds), pp. 159–166.
Oxford: Clarendon Press.

Chau T. (2001) A review of analytical techniques for gait data. Part 1: fuzzy,
statistical and fractal methods. *Gait and Posture* **13**: 49–66.

Chong KC, Vojnic CD, Quanbury AO, Letts RM. (1978) The assessment of the
internal rotation gait in cerebral palsy. *Clinical Orthopaedics and Related
Research* **132**: 145–150.

Chung CY, Stout J, Gage JR. (1997) Rectus femoris transfer – gracilis versus
sartorius. *Gait and Posture* **6**: 137–146.

Cunha UV. (1988) Differential diagnosis of gait disorders in the elderly. *Geriatrics* **43**: 33–42.

Davis RB. (1988) Clinical gait analysis. *IEEE Engineering in Medicine and Biology Magazine* **Sep**: 35–40.

Gage JR. (1983) Gait analysis for decision-making in cerebral palsy. *Bulletin of the Hospital for Joint Diseases Orthopaedic Institute* **43**: 147–163.

Gage JR. (1991) *Gait Analysis in Cerebral Palsy.* London: MacKeith Press.

Gage JR. (1994) Clinical use of kinetics for gait pathology in cerebral palsy (abstract). *Gait and Posture* **2**: 36–37.

Gage JR, Fabian D, Hicks R, Tashman S. (1984) Pre- and postoperative gait analysis in patients with spastic diplegia: a preliminary report. *Journal of Pediatric Orthopedics* **4**: 715–725.

Gage JR, Perry J, Hicks RR et al. (1987) Rectus femoris transfer to improve knee function of children with cerebral palsy. *Developmental Medicine and Child Neurology* **29**: 159–166.

Graham HK, Aoki KR, Autti-Rämö I et al. (2000) Recommendations for the use of botulinum toxin type A in the management of cerebral palsy. *Gait and Posture* **11**: 67–79.

Harrington ED, Lin RS, Gage JR. (1984) Use of the anterior floor reaction orthosis in patients with cerebral palsy. *Orthotics and Prosthetics* **37**: 34–42.

Hicks R, Tashman S, Cary JM et al. (1985) Swing phase control with knee friction in juvenile amputees. *Journal of Orthopaedic Research* **3**: 198–201.

Hicks R, Durinick N, Gage JR. (1988) Differentiation of idiopathic toe-walking and cerebral palsy. *Journal of Pediatric Orthopedics* **8**: 160–163.

Jefferson RJ, Whittle MW. (1989) Biomechanical assessment of unicompartmental knee arthroplasty, total condylar arthroplasty and tibial osteotomy. *Clinical Biomechanics* **4**: 232–242.

Lehmann JF, Condon SM, Price R, deLateur BJ. (1987) Gait abnormalities in hemiplegia: their correction by ankle–foot orthoses. *Archives of Physical Medicine and Rehabilitation* **68**: 763–771.

Lin C-J, Guo L-Y, Su F-C et al. (2000) Common abnormal kinetic patterns of the knee in gait in spastic diplegia of cerebral palsy. *Gait and Posture* **11**: 224–232.

Lord M, Reynolds DP, Hughes JR. (1986) Foot pressure measurement: a review of clinical findings. *Journal of Biomedical Engineering* **8**: 283–294.

New York University (1986) *Lower Limb Orthotics.* New York: Prosthetics and Orthotics, New York University Postgraduate Medical School.

Õunpuu S, Davis RB, DeLuca PA. (1996) Joint kinetics: methods, interpretation and treatment decision-making in children with cerebral palsy and myelomeningocele. *Gait and Posture* **4**: 62–78.

Perry J. (1987) Distal rectus femoris transfer. *Developmental Medicine and Child Neurology* **29**: 153–158.

Perry J. (1992) *Gait Analysis: Normal and Pathological Function.* Thorofare, NJ: SLACK Incorporated.

Prodromos CC, Andriacchi TP, Galante JO. (1985) A relationship between gait and clinical changes following high tibial osteotomy. *Journal of Bone and Joint Surgery* **67A**: 1188–1194.

Roberts CS, Rash GS, Honaker JT et al. (1999) A deficient anterior cruciate ligament does not lead to quadriceps avoidance gait. *Gait and Posture* **10**: 189–199.

Rose GK. (1983) Clinical gait assessment: a personal view. *Journal of Medical Engineering and Technology* **7**: 273–279.

Sutherland DH. (1990) Gait analysis in neuromuscular diseases. *American Academy of Orthopaedic Surgeons: Instructional Course Lectures* **39**: 333–341.

Tashman S, Hicks R, Jendrzejczyk DJ. (1985) Evaluation of a prosthetic shank with variable inertial properties. *Clinical Prosthetics and Orthotics* **9**: 23–28.

Walsh HPJ, Õunpuu S, DeLuca P *et al.* (1993) Effects of bilateral femoral derotation osteotomies on gait in children with cerebral palsy (abstract). *Gait and Posture* **1**: 122.

Waters RL, Garland DE, Perry J *et al.* (1979) Stiff-legged gait in hemiplegia: surgical correction. *Journal of Bone and Joint Surgery* **61A**: 927–933.

Winter DA. (1985) Concerning the scientific basis for the diagnosis of pathological gait and for rehabilitation protocols. *Physiotherapy Canada* **37**: 245–252.

Winters TF, Gage JR, Hicks R. (1987) Gait patterns in spastic hemiplegia in children and young adults. *Journal of Bone and Joint Surgery* **69A**: 437–441.

Case study: gait analysis of a patient

by Karen Hood MS, PT

To illustrate the process of scientific gait analysis, and some of the uses of gait analysis data, a case study will be now be presented. Much of the literature on clinical gait analysis is devoted to the management of cerebral palsy, but the following case illustrates the use of gait analysis in another field – an orthopedic disorder. The process of clinical decision making followed the pattern outlined in Chapter 5: after referral by a physician, a clinical history was obtained, and physical examinations were performed, both by a physician (a specialist in physical medicine) and by a physical therapist. The physical therapy evaluation included range of motion, muscle extensibility and strength, as well as more detailed foot measurements, tone assessment and specific balance tests. Additional measurements were taken for use by the biomechanical modeling software – height, weight, leg length, knee width and ankle width. The subject was videotaped while walking, from both sides, front and back, and was then instrumented with reflective markers for data collection by the television/computer system. It was not deemed appropriate in this case to collect electromyographic data.

The patient, Mr J.B., was 40 years old, and had been referred by his orthopedic surgeon. He had received a crush injury to both feet as a result of an industrial accident 2 years prior to his being referred for gait analysis. His right foot had been treated soon after the accident by open reduction and internal fixation of several metatarsals and phalanges; his left foot had not undergone surgery. He was prescribed custom-made orthotic insoles for both feet, following which his pain eased and his ability to walk improved for 6–8 months. However, since then the symptoms in the left foot had gradually increased. Complaints at the time of the gait analysis included pain and abnormal sensation during walking and in response to moderate pressure, primarily in the left foot. He was referred for gait analysis to explore further treatment options.

Mr J.B. was studied in a laboratory with a six-camera Vicon system and two force platforms (Fig. 4.13). Several practice walks were performed to achieve a natural walking pattern, in which a 'clean' record of a single foot placement was obtained on each force platform. After a single trial with the patient standing, three walking trials were obtained with the patient barefoot, and a further three with him wearing his normal shoes. The patient then left the laboratory. After the data had been processed, the gait laboratory team met to examine and interpret all of the information collected (history, physician and physical therapist examinations, general gait parameters, visual gait analysis, joint angles, moments and powers). A written report, including recommendations for treatment, was supplied to the referring physician.

Physical therapy evaluation

The physical therapy evaluation results are presented in Tables 6.1 and 6.2. To summarize, the passive range of left hip flexion was painful at 90° and internal rotation was limited bilaterally, although it was more limited on the left than the right. Ankle dorsiflexion was limited bilaterally, although more on the left than the right, with the knees both flexed and extended. Hamstring extensibility was decreased bilaterally. Muscle grades of 4/5 (4 points out of a possible 5, by manual muscle testing) were recorded for both hip extensors, left knee flexors, left forefoot inverters and everters, and left ankle dorsiflexors (within the limits set by pain). The patient was unable to perform standing heel raises to test the plantarflexors on the left side, due to pain.

The left first ray was rigid, the right first ray was semi-rigid. Relaxed calcaneal stance position was inverted on the left, and everted on the right. Observation also revealed decreased weight-bearing of the medial aspect of

Table 6.1 Physical therapy assessment of subject J.B.: range of motion and strength

		Range of motion		Strength	
		Right	Left	Right	Left
Hip	flexion	Full	90°*	5/5	4+/5
	extension	10°	10°	4/5	4/5
	abduction	25°	35°	4+/5	4+/5
	internal rotation	0°	10° ER	5/5	5/5
	external rotation	45°	45°	4+/5	4+/5
Knee	extension	5° flexion	5° flexion	5/5	5/5
	flexion	Full	Full	4+/5	4/5
Ankle	dorsiflexion: knee @ 0°	0°	3° pflex	5/5	4/5*
	dorsiflexion: knee @ 90°	5°	0°	–	–
	plantarflexion	60°	60°	5/5	at least 3/5†
Forefoot	inversion	25°	20°	5/5	4/5
	eversion	30°	12°	5/5	4/5
Hindfoot	inversion	–	30°		
	eversion	–	8°		

* within limits of pain
† increased pain after one full heel rise in standing
Full = within functional limits
ER = external rotation
pflex = plantarflexion

Table 6.2 Physical therapy assessment of subject J.B.: muscle extensibility and static alignment measures

Muscle extensibility/static alignment	Right	Left
Hamstrings (popliteal angle)	50°	55°
Thomas test	2°	5°
Leg length (mm)	1020	1000
Malleolar angle	10°	10°
Subtalar neutral	4° varus	4° varus
Foot alignment:		
toes 2–5	5° varus	5° varus
toes 1–5	6° varus	0° varus
Forefoot abduction/adduction	5° adduction	0°
Relaxed calcaneal stance	5° eversion	5° inversion

Joint mobility: Semi-rigid first ray on the right. Rigid first ray on the left.

the left foot, with no contact being made by the great toe. There was little subcutaneous padding on the plantar aspect of the first metatarsal head on the left. Palpation was painful over the plantar aspect of the first and second metatarsal heads on the left foot. Sensation was decreased to light touch on the dorsum of the left foot and the first four toes.

Visual gait analysis

Videotapes were made from each side, and from the front and back, while Mr J.B. walked first barefoot, then wearing shoes with orthotic insoles. Barefoot, observing from the front and back, he was noted, on the left side, to bear weight primarily on the lateral border of the foot. He displayed inversion of the left foot in terminal swing, decreased stance time on the left, and bilateral pes planus. The left great toe was held in extension off the floor. The right calcaneus was everted in stance, the left calcaneus maintained an inverted-to-neutral position in stance. Viewing from both sides, the decreased stance time on the left was again noted, as well as decreased knee extension bilaterally. Trunk posture displayed an increased lumbar lordosis, forward inclination of the head and shoulders, and a minimally increased thoracic kyphosis. With shoes and orthotics, viewing from the front and back, weight was shifted onto the medial border of the left foot, although great toe and calcaneal position could not be determined. Viewing from the side, when compared with the barefoot condition there was a considerable improvement in timing, stability in stance, and overall symmetry.

General gait parameters

Fig. 6.1 and Table 6.3 show the general gait parameters while walking barefoot, and while walking with shoes and orthotic insoles. In

Figure 6.1 General gait parameters during walking; barefoot and with shoes and orthotics.

Table 6.3 General gait parameters of subject J.B. under two conditions: walking barefoot, and walking in shoes with orthotic insoles

	Barefoot	*Shoes + orthotics*	*Normal range*
Cadence (steps/min)	111	100	91–135
Stride length (m)	1.11	1.39	1.25–1.85
Speed (m/s)	1.02	1.16	1.1–1.82
Step length ratio L : R	54 : 46	45 : 55	Approx. 50 : 50
Stance duration L : R	57% : 68%	63% : 64%	Approx. 62% : 62%

summary, Mr J.B.'s cadence was within normal limits under both conditions. Stride length was about 70 per cent of normal barefoot, and within normal limits with shoes and orthotics. When walking barefoot, he had a short right step length and increased right stance phase duration. These two parameters are consistent with an antalgic pattern: the patient is in pain when taking weight on the left foot, so he reduces the duration of the left single support phase. Since the left single support phase corresponds to the right swing phase, there is less time for the right foot to advance during its swing phase, which in turn reduces the right step length. With shoes and orthotics, stance phase durations on both sides were almost the same and approached normal values. The step length was now somewhat greater on the right side, which was probably related to the greater degree of hip flexion on that side.

Figure 6.2 Knee kinematics in the sagittal plane. Left side is represented by a solid line, right side by a dashed line. The three dotted lines represent the normal range (95 per cent confidence interval).

Kinetic and kinematic analysis

The following description is intended to assist the reader in interpreting the charts. Fig. 6.2 presents a typical kinematic chart of the knee angle in the sagittal plane. A solid black line represents the left side; the right side is a dashed line. The normal range (95 per cent confidence limits) is represented by dotted lines. A horizontal axis runs from 0 per cent of the gait cycle to 100 per cent of the cycle (initial contact to next initial contact); the left-hand side of the chart is the stance phase, the right hand, the swing phase. The vertical line shows the division between stance and swing. The small marks at the top of the chart indicate where toe off and initial contact occur on the opposite side.

Kinematics of the pelvis (Fig. 6.3)

Sagittal plane (pelvic tilt): There was an increased anterior pelvic tilt of about 20° throughout the gait cycle, with no significant difference between the barefoot and shoe/orthotic conditions.

Frontal plane (pelvic obliquity): When walking barefoot, the left side of the pelvis was higher than the right side throughout the cycle, indicated by the

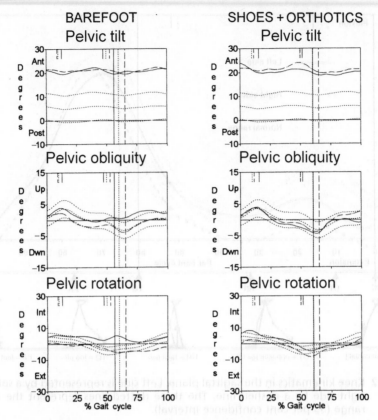

Figure 6.3 Kinematics of pelvis; barefoot and in shoes with orthotics. Pelvic tilt = sagittal plane; pelvic obliquity = frontal plane; pelvic rotation = transverse plane.

solid line being above the dashed line in the chart. With shoes, the two sides were equal for most of the cycle, and were within the normal range.

Transverse plane (pelvic rotation): In both conditions the left side of the pelvis was more anterior than the right, represented on the chart as an 'internal rotation' on the left and an 'external rotation' on the right. The overall range of excursion, however, approximated normal ranges under both conditions.

Sagittal plane kinematics of the hip, knee and ankle (Fig. 6.4)

Hip: In both conditions hip motion was biased into flexion, due to a reduction in extension, with a total range of motion that was less than the normal range. The increased hip flexion was related to the previously noted increased anterior pelvic tilt, as described in Chapter 3 (increased lumbar lordosis).

Knee: When walking barefoot, there was a bilateral reduction in both stance phase and swing phase knee flexion. When walking with shoes and orthotics, swing phase knee flexion increased bilaterally, and stance phase flexion increased on the left, but not the right.

Figure 6.4 Kinematics of hip, knee and ankle in the sagittal plane; barefoot and in shoes with orthotics. Flx = flexion; Ext = extension; Dor = dorsiflexion; Pla = plantarflexion.

Ankle: Barefoot, there was a significant reduction in ankle plantarflexion before, during, and immediately after toe off, bilaterally. With shoes and orthotics, ankle plantarflexion improved on both sides.

Normal ankle kinematics and kinetics (Fig. 6.5)

The ankle kinematics, moments and powers from normal subjects are illustrated in Fig. 6.5. The charts show the internal joint moments, which oppose the moments generated by external forces. Internal moments may be generated actively, by contraction of muscles, or passively, by ligaments coming under tension.

As the ankle progressively dorsiflexes, between 10 per cent and 50 per cent of the gait cycle, the internal plantarflexion moment increases through eccentric contraction of the ankle plantarflexors, possibly augmented by the stretching of elastic tissues. The power curve confirms this by indicating power absorption during this phase. Between 50 per cent and 60 per cent of the gait cycle, the ankle plantarflexes, the internal joint moment being produced by concentric contraction of the plantarflexors. This is also

Figure 6.5 Normal values for ankle kinematics, moments and powers.

Figure 6.6 Ankle kinematics, moments and powers in the sagittal plane; barefoot and in shoes with orthotics. Gen = generation; Abs = absorption.

confirmed by the power curve, which shows an abrupt burst of power generation.

Ankle kinematics and kinetics in Mr J.B. (Fig. 6.6)

Ankle moment: In both barefoot and shoe/orthotic conditions, the ankle moment on the right side was within the normal range. On the left, there was a normal ankle moment when walking in shoes with orthotics, but in the barefoot condition the (internal) plantarflexor moment was reduced, suggesting a reluctance to take weight on the forefoot. The previous findings of decreased left stance phase duration and decreased ankle plantarflexion during pre-swing further support a tendency to avoid weight transfer to the forefoot.

Ankle power: When walking barefoot, the power absorption in terminal stance was increased bilaterally in comparison with normal ranges. Power generation, however, was markedly reduced on the right, and nearly absent on the left. With shoes and orthotics, the ankle power curves approximated normal ranges. Since both the ankle moment and kinematics improved in the shoe/orthotic condition, it was to be expected that the joint power would also have improved, as joint power is the product of the joint moment and the joint angular velocity. Deviations from normal which were still present in the shoe/orthotic condition included exaggerated power absorption in terminal stance bilaterally (due possibly to the decreased ankle range of motion and increased muscular tightness noted during the clinical exam), and a slightly reduced power generation on the left.

Summary of findings

1. When walking barefoot, there was a marked antalgic pattern, with reduced stance phase duration on the left and reduced right step length. Weight-bearing was primarily on the lateral border of the foot. On the left there was also an extended first ray, limited ankle sagittal plane movement, and a reduction of power generation just prior to toe off.
2. The use of shoes and orthotic insoles eliminated the antalgic timing pattern, and improved the sagittal plane ankle motion bilaterally.
3. Both when walking barefoot and in shoes and orthotics, there was an exaggerated anterior pelvic tilt and reduced sagittal plane hip motion, with a reduction in the range of hip extension. Sagittal plane knee motion, especially during swing, improved with shoes and orthotics. When walking barefoot, ankle plantarflexion was decreased on both sides, left worse than right, during pre-swing and initial swing. When walking with shoes and insoles, the ankle motion was approximately normal.
4. Kinetic analysis showed a marked reduction in power generation at the ankles during pre-swing when walking barefoot, especially on the left. With shoes and orthotics, ankle power curves improved significantly, although power generation on the left remained less than that on the right. This increased plantarflexor power generation just before toe off probably increased the rate at which the knee flexed, and thereby improved swing phase knee flexion.

Recommendations

1. While the orthotics significantly improved the gait pattern, the patient continued to present with some pain during ambulation. Therefore his orthotic prescription needed to be reviewed carefully, to address the need for protection of the plantar surface, with preservation of foot dynamics.
2. The limited dorsiflexion noted on static examination, combined with the increased power absorption in terminal stance, should be addressed by an exercise program to stretch the triceps surae bilaterally. Increased dorsiflexion at the talocrural joint may also assist to decrease excessive loading to the forefoot during stance.

7

Gait analysis data on CD-ROM

This textbook is accompanied by a CD-ROM, which is designed to give the reader access to some 'real' gait data, both from a normal subject and from a patient with cerebral palsy. The data were collected using the Vicon system, and the multimedia presentation was prepared using the powerful Polygon program. The CD-ROM includes Polygon Viewer, which is used to view reports made using the Polygon Authoring Tool. Both Vicon and Polygon are products of Vicon Motion Systems Ltd.

This CD should run on any computer with the Windows 98 (or later) operating system and a CD-ROM drive. A suggested minimum configuration for a satisfactory display is a 250 MHz processor and 64 MB of RAM. On older or less well-equipped machines, the program may not run at all, or the display may be jerky and incomplete.

If the autorun facility has been enabled on the computer, the Polygon Viewer program should start automatically after the CD-ROM has been inserted. If this does not happen, there are two possible ways to start the program:

1. Use Windows Explorer to navigate to the CD drive (usually D:) and double-click on 'PolygonViewer.exe'
2. Click on the 'Start' icon, select 'Run...', type in 'D:PolygonViewer' (without spaces, and without quotation marks), and press the Enter key. If the CD drive is not D:, substitute it's name in the command.

The CD contains the following items:

1. Brief instructions on using Polygon Viewer
2. A normal subject walking
3. A child with cerebral palsy walking (pre- and post-operative).

Sincere thanks are given to the following, who have made this CD possible:

1. James Carollo and Nancy Denniston from the Center for Gait and Movement Analysis (CGMA) at The Children's Hospital, Denver, for providing the data from the normal subject and the patient

2. Vicon Motion Systems Ltd, for allowing the author to use their Polygon Authoring Tool software. They may be found on the Internet at http://www.vicon.com/, or contacted as follows:

Head Office: Vicon Motion Systems Ltd, 14 Minns Business Park, West Way, Oxford OX2 0JB, England.
Tel: +44 0 1865 261800
Fax: +44 0 1865 240527
Email: sales@vicon.com

In USA: Vicon Motion Systems, 9 Spectrum Pointe Drive, Lake Forest, CA 92630. Tel: (1) 949 472 9140
Fax: (1) 949 472 9136
Email: sales@vicon.com.

Appendix 1

Normal ranges for gait parameters

Approximate range (95 per cent limits) for general gait parameters in free-speed walking by normal FEMALE subjects of different ages

Age (years)	Cadence (steps/min)	Cycle time (s)	Stride length (m)	Speed (m/s)
13–14	103–150	0.80–1.17	0.99–1.55	0.90–1.62
15–17	100–144	0.83–1.20	1.03–1.57	0.92–1.64
18–49	98–138	0.87–1.22	1.06–1.58	0.94–1.66
50–64	97–137	0.88–1.24	1.04–1.56	0.91–1.63
65–80	96–136	0.88–1.25	0.94–1.46	0.80–1.52

Approximate range (95 per cent limits) for general gait parameters in free-speed walking by normal MALE subjects of different ages

Age (years)	Cadence (steps/min)	Cycle time (s)	Stride length (m)	Speed (m/s)
13–14	100–149	0.81–1.20	1.06–1.64	0.95–1.67
15–17	96–142	0.85–1.25	1.15–1.75	1.03–1.75
18–49	91–135	0.89–1.32	1.25–1.85	1.10–1.82
50–64	82–126	0.95–1.46	1.22–1.82	0.96–1.68
65–80	81–125	0.96–1.48	1.11–1.71	0.81–1.61

Approximate range (95 per cent limits) for general gait parameters in free-speed walking by normal CHILDREN of different ages (ages 1–7 years based on Sutherland *et al.*, 1988)

Age (years)	Cadence (steps/min)	Cycle time (s)	Stride length (m)	Speed (m/s)
1	127–223	0.54–0.94	0.29–0.58	0.32–0.96
1.5	126–212	0.57–0.95	0.33–0.66	0.39–1.03
2	125–201	0.60–0.96	0.37–0.73	0.45–1.09
2.5	124–190	0.63–0.97	0.42–0.81	0.52–1.16
3	123–188	0.64–0.98	0.46–0.89	0.58–1.22
3.5	122–186	0.65–0.98	0.50–0.96	0.65–1.29
4	121–184	0.65–0.99	0.54–1.04	0.67–1.32
5	119–180	0.67–1.01	0.59–1.10	0.71–1.37
6	117–176	0.68–1.03	0.64–1.16	0.75–1.43
7	115–172	0.70–1.04	0.69–1.22	0.80–1.48
8	113–169	0.71–1.06	0.75–1.30	0.82–1.50
9	111–166	0.72–1.08	0.82–1.37	0.83–1.53

Appendix 2

Conversions between measurement units

For each variable, the Système International d'Unités (SI) uses a funda-mental unit and a series of multiples and submultiples, in steps of 10^3, as follows:

pico (p) 10^{-12} kilo (k) 10^3
nano (n) 10^{-9} mega (M) 10^6
micro (µ) 10^{-6} giga (G) 10^9
milli (m) 10^{-3} tera (T) 10^{12}

Length

SI units: millimeter (mm), meter (m), kilometer (km)
Other units: inch (in), foot (ft), mile (mi)

1 mm = 0.039370 in
1 m = 1000 mm = 39.370 in = 3.2808 ft
1 km = 1000 m = 0.62137 mi

Area

SI unit: square millimeter (mm^2), square meter (m^2)
Other units: square inch (in^2), square foot (ft^2)

$1 mm^2 = 0.0015500 in^2$
$1 m^2 = 10^6 mm^2 = 10.764 ft^2$

Volume

SI units: cubic millimeter (mm^3), cubic meter (m^3)
Other units: milliliter (ml), liter (l), cubic inch (in^3), cubic foot (ft^3), fluid ounce (fl oz), gallon (gal)

$1 ml = 1000 mm^3 = 0.061024 in^3$
1 l = 1000 ml = 35.195 fl oz (UK) = 33.814 fl oz (US)
$1 m^3 = 1000 l = 219.97 gal (UK) = 264.17 gal (US) = 35.315 ft^3$

Linear velocity

SI unit: meter per second (m/s or m s^{-1})
Other units: feet per second (ft/s or ft s^{-1}), kilometers per hour (kph), miles per hour (mph)

1 m/s $= 3.2808$ ft/s $= 3.6000$ kph $= 2.2369$ mph

Linear acceleration

SI unit: meter per second per second (m/s^2 or m s^{-2})
Other units: feet per second per second (ft/s^2 or ft s^{-2})

1 m/s$^2 = 3.2808$ ft/s^2

Acceleration due to gravity

$g = 9.80665$ m s^{-2} $= 32.174$ ft s^{-2}

Mass

SI units: gram (g), kilogram (kg)
Other units: ounce (oz), pound (lb), slug

1 g $= 0.035274$ oz
1 kg $= 1000$ g $= 2.2046$ lb $= 0.068522$ slug

Force

SI unit: newton (N) (equivalent to kg m/s^2)
Other units: dyne (dyn), kilogram force (kgf), kilopond (kp) – identical to kilogram force, pound force (lbf), poundal (pdl)

1 N $= 10^5$ dyn $= 0.10197$ kgf $= 0.22481$ lbf $= 7.2330$ pdl

Pressure and stress

SI units: pascal (Pa), kilopascal (kPa), megapascal (MPa)
Other units: bar, millimeter of mercury (mm Hg), inch of water (in H$_2$O), physical atmosphere (atm), pound force per square inch (psi), kilogram force per square centimeter (kgf/cm^2)

1 Pa $= 1$ Nm^{-2} $= 10^{-5}$ bar
1 kPa $= 1000$ Pa $= 4.0146$ in H$_2$O $= 7.5006$ mm Hg
1 MPa $= 1000$ kPa $= 9.8692$ atm $= 145.04$ psi $= 10.197$ kgf/cm^2

Energy

SI units: joule (J), kilojoule (kJ), megajoule (MJ)
Other units: erg, 15° calorie, 15° kilocalorie ($kcal_{15}$) – identical to Calorie, used in dietary calculations – British thermal unit (Btu), kilowatt hour (kWh)

$1 J = 10^7 \, erg = 0.23892 \, cal_{15}$
$1 \, kJ = 1000 J = 0.23892 \, kcal_{15} = 0.94781 \, Btu$
$1 \, MJ = 1000 \, kJ = 0.27778 \, kWh$

Power

SI units: watt (W), kilowatt (kW)
Other unit: horsepower (hp)

$1 W = 1 J s^{-1}$
$1 \, kW = 1.3410 \, hp$

Plane angle

SI unit: radian (rad)
Other unit: degree (°)

$180° = \pi \, rad$
$1 \, rad = 180/\pi = 57.296° \quad 1° = 0.017453 \, rad$

Appendix 3

Sources of further information

Journal articles

Papers in the scientific journals constitute the major repository for knowledge on any scientific subject, including gait analysis. A number of key papers are cited as references in this book. A computer search of the Medline database, using suitable keywords, will uncover many more. As well as its availability through research libraries, it is also possible to access Medline on the Internet, through the PubMed service (http://www.ncbi.nlm.nih.gov/PubMed/).

Papers on gait analysis are most frequently found in the following journals, although a large number of other journals also contain occasional papers on the subject:

Clinical Biomechanics
Clinical Orthopaedics and Related Research
Gait and Posture
Journal of Biomechanics
Journal of Biomedical Engineering
Journal of Bone and Joint Surgery
Physical Therapy

Another convenient way to find references to gait analysis topics is to use the bibliographic database developed by Christopher Vaughan and colleagues, which is on the CD-ROM named GaitCD, listed below under 'Computer Programs'.

Learned societies

There are a number of learned societies which focus on gait analysis and related subjects, including the Gait and Clinical Movement Analysis Society (GCMAS), the International Society for Postural and Gait Research (ISPG), the European Society of Movement Analysis in Adults and Children (ESMAC), and the Società Italiana di Analisi del Movimento in Clinica (SIAMOC). An even greater number of societies include gait analysis among their interests, including the International Society of Biomechanics (ISB) and the various national and regional societies of biomechanics. Up-to-date information on these societies will be found on the Internet (see below).

Conferences and conference proceedings

The most up-to-date information on gait analysis research will always be found in the oral and poster presentations at relevant conferences. The conferences with the highest content of gait analysis research are those run by the organizations listed in the preceding section. Details of forth-coming conferences will be found in the calendar sections of some of the journals, and on the Internet (see below). Many conferences publish books of proceedings or abstracts, which are available for purchase. Few libraries have these books, and it usually necessary to contact the conference orga-nizers to obtain them. Exceptions to this are the GCMAS, ESMAC and SIAMOC meetings, the abstracts from which are published in the journal *Gait and Posture*.

Textbooks

Each of the chapters in this book ends in a bibliography, which lists some major texts providing further information on the topics covered by the chapter.

Videotapes

A number of individuals and institutions have developed videotapes as learning aids for gait analysis. Those the author is aware of are as follows:

Physical Examination of the Musculoskeletal System, Program 9: Gait by Larry B. Conochie
American Academy of Orthopaedic Surgeons
222 South Prospect Avenue
Park Ridge, Illinois 60068, USA

Normal Development of Walking by Janet L. Hale
Therapy Skill Builders
3830 E. Bellevue
P.O. Box 42050
Tucson, Arizona 85733, USA

Observation of Human Gait (in three parts)
Health Sciences Media Services 0J1 WMC
University of Alberta
Edmonton, Alberta T6G 2R7 Canada

Normal Walking
Gillette Children's Hospital
200 East University Avenue
St Paul, Minnesota 55101, USA
Telephone: +1-612-291-2848

Principles of Pathologic Gait in Cerebral Palsy
Gillette Children's Hospital (address as above).

Running and Sprinting: A Dynamic Analysis
Gillette Children's Hospital (address as above).

Several other videos on gait are available from:

Los Amigos Research and Education Institute, Inc.
P.O. Box 3500
12841 Dahlia St., Bldg. #306
Downey, California 90242, USA

Computer programs

The following computer programs are also likely to be useful for learning about gait and gait analysis:

GaitCD (CD-ROM, for IBM-PC running Windows 95 or later)
Christopher L. Vaughan (1999)
Kiboho Publishers
P.O. Box 769
Howard Place
Western Cape 7450
South Africa

Normal Walking (CD-ROM, for IBM-PC or Macintosh)
Gillette Children's Hospital (address in 'Videotapes' above)

Principles of Pathologic Gait in Cerebral Palsy (CD-ROM, for IBM-PC or Macintosh)
Gillette Children's Hospital (address in 'Videotapes' above).

BioWare Force Platform Analysis Software (for IBM-PC)
Kistler Instrumente AG Winterthur
P.O. Box 304
CH-8408 Winterthur
Switzerland

The Internet

The Internet is changing extremely rapidly. The information below is current at the time of publication, but may be somewhat out-of-date by the time you read this!

Probably the most useful resource is the Clinical Gait Analysis website (http://guardian.curtin.edu.au/cga/)

A great deal of information on gait analysis can be also found on the biomechanics 'list', known as BIOMCH-L (http://isb.ri.ccf.org/biomch-l/index.html/)

Some information about gait analysis is included in the Kinesiology and Biomechanics Teacher's Resource Page (http://www.usfca.edu/ess/resourcepage.htm/)

Many other Internet sites contain information relevant to gait analysis, which can be found by entering suitable keywords into one of the many search engines. Further information is available from the many books about the Internet, or from the providers of the on-line services.

Glossary

Abduction – movement of a limb away from the midline, in the frontal plane

Adduction – movement of a limb towards the midline, in the frontal plane

Afferent – nerves or nerve impulses reaching the central nervous system from peripheral parts of the body

Aiming – walking in an unnatural way, so that the foot will land in a particular position, e.g. on a force platform

Anatomical position – used for anatomical descriptions: standing upright, with the feet together, the arms by the sides and the palms forward

Ankylosis – destruction of a joint, either by surgery or disease, resulting in a total loss of movement

Antagonists – muscles with opposing actions, e.g. flexion *versus* extension

Anterior – to the front of the body (in the anatomical position)

Ataxia – loss of coordination, due to disease of the central nervous system

Athetosis – disorder of the central nervous system, resulting in continual uncoordinated movements of the limbs

Atrophy – loss of bulk, especially of a muscle

Baclofen – a drug used to reduce muscle tone

Biofeedback – allowing a person to see how well they are performing a task, so that they can make immediate improvements

Botulinum toxin – used by injection to paralyze muscles; the effects generally last about 3 months

Bunion – see *hallux valgus*

Butterfly diagram – method of displaying ground reaction force data

Cadence – the number of steps (not strides) in a given time, usually 1 minute

Calliper – orthosis (q.v.) fitted around one or both legs, to compensate for weakness or paralysis; also spelled 'caliper'

Caudad – towards the 'tail'; equivalent of inferior

Center of gravity – in mechanical calculations, the point within an object at which it can be assumed that the mass of the object is concentrated

Central pattern generator – networks of neurons (q.v.) in the brain and spinal cord which act together to generate repetitive motions, such as walking

Center of pressure – the point beneath the foot through which it can be assumed that the ground reaction force is passing

Cerebellar ataxia – ataxia (q.v.) due to disease of the cerebellum

Cerebrovascular accident (CVA) – brain damage due to blood clot or hemorrhage; also known as 'stroke'

Cephalad – towards the head; equivalent of superior

Cerebral palsy (CP) – neurological disorder with spasticity (q.v.) and incoordination, caused by brain damage around the time of birth

Clonus – jerky contraction of a muscle, usually due to spasticity (q.v.)

Co-contraction – when two different muscles contract at the same time

Concentric contraction – muscle contraction in which the muscle gets shorter as it develops tension

Congenital dislocation of hip (CDH) – condition present at birth in which the head of femur is not properly contained in the acetabulum

Contracture – reduction in the range of motion of a joint, due to restriction by inelastic connective tissue

Coronal plane – see *frontal plane*

Couple – two parallel forces acting in opposite directions, which combine to produce a moment (q.v.)

Coupling – due to the alignment of a joint, movement in one direction automatically produces movement in another direction

Coupled movements – see *coupling*

Coxa vara – abnormal angulation of the upper end of the femur, making the femoral neck too horizontal

Cycle time – the time taken to complete a single gait cycle

Derotation osteotomy – operation in which a long bone is cut through and held in a partially rotated position while it heals

Determinants of gait – six strategies used to minimize energy consumption in normal gait

Diabetes – disease in which control of blood sugar is imperfect through lack of, or abnormal response to, the hormone insulin

Diabetic neuropathy – loss of function of peripheral nerves, especially sensory nerves in the feet, due to diabetes (q.v.)

Diplegia – paralysis of both arms or both legs

Distal – away from the rest of the body

Deep – far from the surface

Dorsal – the posterior surface

Dorsal rhizotomy – selective cutting of some of the sensory fibers in the posterior (dorsal) root of a number of spinal nerves; used to reduce spasticity, by interfering with the stretch reflex

Dorsiflexion – movement of the foot towards the knee

Dorsum – the back of the hand, or the upper surface of the foot

Double pendulum – a structure that is suspended at its top end, but jointed in the middle; it can swing like a pendulum about both joints

Double support – period in the gait cycle in which both feet are on the ground, one in loading response and one in pre-swing

Eccentric contraction – muscle contraction in which the external force overpowers the muscle so that it gets longer

Efferent – nerves or nerve impulses leaving the central nervous system, directed towards peripheral parts of the body

Electrogoniometer – device that fixes across a joint and puts out a continuous electrical signal describing joint angle

Electromyogram (EMG) – recording of the electrical activity of a muscle

Evert, eversion – internal rotation about the long axis of the foot

Extension – sagittal plane movement at a joint, the distal segment usually moving posteriorly (anteriorly at the knee)

External moment – moment applied from outside, as by an external force which is attempting to flex or extend a joint

External rotation – rotation of a limb about its long axis, the anterior surface moving laterally

Extrapyramidal system – areas of the brain and spinal cord providing coordination and control, as opposed to direct activation of muscles

Feet adjacent – event in the swing phase of the gait cycle when the foot of the swinging leg passes the supporting foot

Flexion – sagittal plane movement at a joint, the distal segment usually moving anteriorly (posteriorly at the knee)

Flexion contracture – deformity in which contraction of soft tissues prevents a joint from extending fully

Foot flat – point in the stance phase of the gait cycle at which the forefoot contacts the ground, when initial contact has been made by the heel

Foot slap – abrupt and audible lowering of the foot following initial contact (q.v.)

Footstrike – see *initial contact*

Force platform, forceplate – common piece of gait analysis equipment, for measuring the ground reaction force (q.v.).

Forefoot – the five metatarsal bones and the toes

Frontal plane – divides a body part into front and back portions

Gait – the manner or style of walking

Gait cycle – the time interval between two successive occurrences of one of the repetitive events of walking (usually initial contact on one side)

Ground reaction force – the upward force applied by the ground to the foot, in response to the downward force applied by the foot to the ground; commonly measured by force platforms

Hallux – the big toe, or great toe

Hallux valgus – deformity affecting the big toe, in which the metatarso-phalangeal joint is in valgus; also known as bunion

Hansen's disease – bacterial infection causing progressive destruction of nerves and sensory loss; also known as leprosy

Heel rise – event in the stance phase of the gait cycle at which the heel lifts away from the supporting surface

Heelstrike – a distinct impact between the heel and the ground at initial contact

Hemiparesis – partial paralysis affecting one side of the body

Hemiplegia – complete paralysis affecting one side of the body, usually due to brain disease or injury

High tibial osteotomy – operation to change the alignment of the upper tibia, to alter the direction of forces acting on the knee

Hindfoot – two bones in the foot: talus and calcaneus

Horizontal plane – see *transverse plane*

Inferior – lower down the body (in the anatomical position)

Initial contact – event in the gait cycle when first contact is made between the foot and ground; made by the heel in normal gait; marks the transition from swing phase to stance phase

Initial swing – period in the swing phase of the gait cycle between toe off and feet adjacent

Internal moment – moment generated by muscles and/or ligaments in the vicinity of a joint

Internal rotation – rotation of a limb about its long axis, the anterior surface moving medially

Intrathecal – injection into the fluid surrounding the spinal cord

Invert, inversion – external rotation about the long axis of the foot

Isometric contraction – muscle contraction in which a muscle develops tension but remains the same length

Lateral – away from the midline of the body

Lateral rotation – see *external rotation*

Lever arm – the perpendicular distance between a force and the axis of rotation, when generating a moment (q.v.)

Line of gravity – a vertical line downwards from the center of gravity (q.v.)

Line of progression – straight line corresponding to the average path taken by the body in walking

Loading response – period in the stance phase of the gait cycle between initial contact and opposite toe off

Lordosis – forward curvature of the spine, causing concavity of the lumbar region of the back

Lower motor neuron – nerve fiber producing muscular contraction, running from the spinal cord to the muscle

Marker – an object fixed to a point on the skin, so that it is visible to an optical measurement system; typically a small sphere covered in reflective tape

Medial – towards the midline of the body

Medial rotation – see *internal rotation*

Median plane – the midline sagittal plane, which divides the whole body into right and left halves

Metatarsalgia – severe pain beneath the metatarsal heads, typically caused by nerve compression

Midfoot – five tarsal bones: navicular, cuboid, and the medial, intermediate and lateral cuneiforms

Mid-stance – period in the stance phase of the gait cycle between opposite toe off and heel rise

Mid-swing – period in the swing phase of the gait cycle between feet adjacent and tibia vertical

Moment, moment of force – a turning effect; typically a force being applied in such a way that it causes a rotation

Moment arm – see *lever arm*

Multiple sclerosis – progressive neurological disease, caused by a patchy loss of myelin from neurons in brain and spinal cord

Muscular dystrophy – progressive wasting disease affecting muscles, usually hereditary

Noise – random errors that affect any form of measurement

Opposite initial contact – event in the stance phase of the gait cycle when the other foot makes initial contact with the ground; occurs at around 50 per cent of the cycle in normal gait

Opposite toe off – event in the stance phase of the gait cycle when the other foot is leaving the ground. Generally close in time to foot flat (q.v.)

Oral – taken by mouth

Orthosis – an external support for some part of the body; also known as a brace

Osteoarthritis – degenerative disease affecting the joints, with pain, stiffness and deformity

Osteotomy – surgical operation involving cutting through a bone; an abnormally rotated bone may be cut through, rotated, and allowed to heal in the new position

Paralysis – loss of the ability voluntarily to contract a muscle

Paraplegia – complete paralysis of the legs, usually due to disease or injury of the spinal cord

Paresis – partial paralysis

Parkinsonism – progressive degenerative neurological condition, involving tremor and weakness; also known as Parkinson's disease

Perineum – the area of skin around the anus and genitalia

Peripheral nerves – nerves which originate in the spinal cord, as opposed to cranial nerves, which originate in the brain

Peripheral neuropathy – loss of function due to degeneration of the nerves of the hands and feet

Physiological cost index (PCI) – method of estimating relative energy consumption using the heart rate

Plane of progression – a flat vertical plane following the average path taken by the body in walking

Plantarflexion – movement of the foot away from the knee

Poliomyelitis – virus disease causing destruction of lower motor neurons, with muscle atrophy and paralysis

Posterior – to the back of the body (in the anatomical position)

Pressure sore – ulcer (q.v.) forming on an area of skin exposed to sufficient pressure to cut off the blood supply

Pre-swing – period in the stance phase of the gait cycle between opposite initial contact and toe off

Pronation – forearm: internal rotation; foot: a combination of eversion, dorsiflexion and forefoot abduction

Proprioception – unconscious feedback on joint position, force in ligaments and tendons, etc.

Prosthetic joint – an artificial joint, implanted in place of the natural joint

Prosthetic limb – an artificial limb, usually fixed onto a stump following amputation

Proximal – towards the rest of the body

Push off – see *pre-swing*

Quadriplegia – paralysis of both arms and both legs; also known as tetraplegia

Rheumatoid arthritis – painful inflammation of the joints, caused by a connective tissue disease

Rhizotomy – see *dorsal rhizotomy*

Rockers – the three mechanisms used to move the tibia forward while the foot is on the ground

Sagittal plane – divides part of the body into right and left portions

Selective dorsal rhizotomy – see *dorsal rhizotomy*

Single support – period during the gait cycle in which only one foot is in contact with the ground; corresponds to swing phase on the other side

Slipped femoral epiphysis – hip disease involving displacement of the articular surface of the femoral head, typically in teenagers

Spasticity – involuntary resistance of muscles to being stretched

Spina bifida – incomplete development of the vertebrae, resulting in damage to the associated spinal cord

Stance phase – that part of the gait cycle for one side in which the foot is on the ground

Stance time – the duration of the stance phase, between initial contact and toe off

Step – the advancement of a single foot

Step length – the distance one foot moves ahead of the other foot during the gait cycle

Step-to, step-through – gait patterns used when walking with crutches

Stride – the advancement of both feet (one step by each side)

Stride length – the distance either foot moves forward during the gait cycle

Stroke – see *cerebrovascular accident*

Subluxation – partial dislocation of a joint, the joint surfaces being able to move in and out of the correct alignment

Subcutaneous – beneath the skin

Superficial – close to the surface

Superior – higher up the body (in the anatomical position)

Supination – forearm: external rotation; foot: inversion, plantarflexion and forefoot adduction

Swing phase – that part of the gait cycle for one side in which the foot is off the ground, moving through the air

Swing time – the duration of the swing phase, between toe off and initial contact

Tabes dorsalis – loss of sensation and proprioception, due to effect of syphilis on the sensory pathways of the spinal cord

Tenotomy – surgical cutting of a tendon, either to free it completely, or to lengthen or shorten it

Terminal stance – period in the stance phase of the gait cycle between heel rise and opposite initial contact

Terminal swing – period in the swing phase of the gait cycle between tibia vertical and the next initial contact

Tetraparesis – partial paralysis affecting all four limbs

Tetraplegia – see *quadriplegia*

Tibia vertical – event in the swing phase of gait in which the tibia passes through the vertical in moving from behind the body to in front of it

Toe drag – failure to clear the ground with the toes during the swing phase of gait

Toe in – the angle between the foot and the line of progression, when the toes are inclined medially

Toe out – the angle between the foot and the line of progression, when the toes are inclined laterally

Toe off – event in the gait cycle when the foot (generally the toe) leaves the ground; marks the transition from the stance phase to the swing phase

Toestrike – making initial contact (q.v.) with the toes, rather than the heel or flat foot

Tone – the amount by which a muscle resists attempts to stretch it: high tone is present in spasticity (q.v.)

Torque – see *moment*

Transection – cutting through completely (applied to spinal cord)

Transfemoral amputation – amputation of a leg between the hip and knee joints

Transtibial amputation – amputation of a leg between the knee and ankle joints

Transverse plane – divides a body part into upper and lower portions

Ulcer – loss of covering skin or epithelium

Upper motor neuron – nerve fiber producing muscular contraction, running from the brain to the spinal cord, where it connects with lower motor neurons

Valgus – joint angulation, with the distal segment sloping away from the midline

Varus – joint angulation, with the distal segment sloping towards the midline

Ventral – the anterior surface

Walking base – the side-to-side distance between the paths taken by the two feet

Index